Bashar A. Aqel, M.D., Julie K. Heimbach, M.D., C. Burcin Taner, M.D.

MAYO CLINIC GUIDE TO ORGAN TRANSPLANT

A guide for patients, caregivers and living donors from the **world's leading transplant experts**

MAYO CLINIC | Press

Medical Editors | Bashar A. Aqel, M.D., Julie K. Heimbach, M.D., C. Burcin Taner, M.D.
Contributors | Thomas M. Dauw, R.Ph., Melodie A. Deis, R.N., C.C.T.C., Jacque L. Gonzales, R.N., Carrie C. Jadlowiec, M.D., Sheila G. Jowsey-Gregoire, M.D., Cassie C. Kennedy, M.D., Parag C. Patel, M.D., Lynn M. Pearson, R.N., C.C.T.C., Mikel Prieto, M.D., Jenna M. Rosenberg, M.S.W., L.M.S.W., Terry D. Schneekloth, M.D., Patti Tait, M.S.N., R.N., Liu Yang, M.B.B.S., Daniel S. Yip, M.D.

Proceeds from the sale of every book benefit important medical research and education at Mayo Clinic.

To stay informed about Mayo Clinic Press, please subscribe to our free e-newsletter at MCPress.MayoClinic.org or follow us on social media.

For bulk sales, contact Mayo Clinic at SpecialSalesMayoBooks@mayo.edu.

Image Credits: All photographs and illustrations are copyright of Mayo Foundation for Medical Education and Research (MFMER) except for the following: Cover / PCH-Vector / iStock / Getty Images Plus

MAYO CLINIC PRESS
200 First St. SW
Rochester, MN 55905
MCPress.MayoClinic.org

ISBN 979-8-88770-394-7 (hardcover)
989-8-88770-395-4 (ebook)

Library of Congress Control Number: 2025017302
Library of Congress Cataloging-in-Publication Data is available upon request.

Printed in China
First printing: 2026

Contents

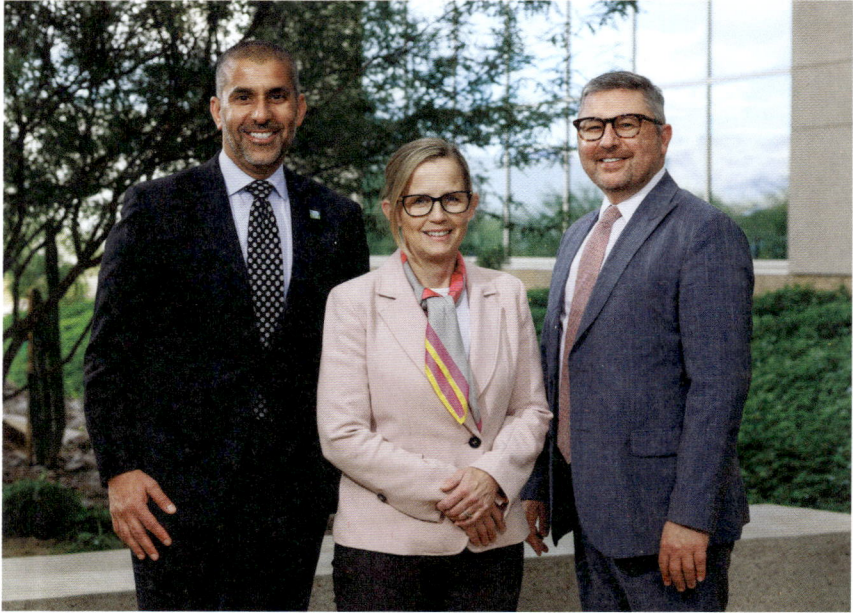

Bashar A. Aqel, M.D., is a gastroenterologist and transplant hepatologist at Mayo Clinic and the director of the Mayo Clinic Transplant Center in Arizona. He also is a professor of medicine at Mayo Clinic College of Medicine and Science. Dr. Aqel's areas of clinical expertise include improved access to liver transplantation, expanding the liver donor pool and care of patients awaiting liver transplant.

Julie K. Heimbach, M.D., is a transplant surgeon at Mayo Clinic and the director of the Mayo Clinic Transplant Center in Minnesota. She also is a professor of surgery at Mayo Clinic College of Medicine and Science. Her primary focus is adult and pediatric liver transplantation and living-donor surgery. Dr. Heimbach is actively involved in transplant research including analysis and treatment outcomes for patients with complex liver transplants and long-term outcomes of living donors.

C. Burcin Taner, M.D., is a transplant surgeon at Mayo Clinic and director of the Mayo Clinic Transplant Center in Florida. He also is a professor of surgery at Mayo Clinic College of Medicine and Science. Dr. Taner's areas of expertise include liver, kidney and pancreas transplantation. He is actively involved in efforts to identify efficient patient care and improve quality of life after transplantation. Dr. Taner is leading Mayo Clinic's innovation efforts in organ failure and transplantation.

Introduction

Organ transplantation is one of the great advances in modern medicine, providing a second chance at life for people of all ages.

As scientists and surgeons embrace new techniques and technologies to recover, preserve and rehabilitate donor organs, more people are receiving transplantation surgery and with greater success. In 2024, a record-setting 48,149 transplants were performed in the United States. Outcomes after transplantation also continue to improve.

While this progress is very encouraging, there's still a critical shortage of available organs for transplant. At any given time, more than 100,000 people are awaiting a transplant in the United States. Many people may experience a long wait to receive a new organ and are at risk of death while they wait. Understanding the need to improve organ availability, transplant specialists are making greater efforts on several fronts to increase organ donation, including encouraging more people to consider becoming living organ donors.

The most common organ transplants are the kidney, heart, lungs, pancreas and liver. However, surgeons are transplanting other organs with increased frequency, including the small intestine, hand, face, larynx and trachea.

Organ transplantation is a complex procedure. It requires a precise diagnosis and a team of experts from a variety of specialties who understand not just the surgery but the underlying health issues making the surgery necessary. And it requires dedicated healthcare staff to ensure a full recovery.

Mayo Clinic is the largest integrated transplant provider in the nation. Every year, more than 150 surgeons and physicians and hundreds of trained staff perform more than 2,000 solid organ transplants at Mayo Clinic's campuses in Arizona, Florida and Minnesota. Mayo Clinic produces some of the best outcomes in the country, including speed to transplant, organ acceptance and patient survival.

With this experience and knowledge, we want to share what we've learned about organ transplantation — before, during and after surgery — to help those who may be on the transplant journey. We wrote this book with these goals in mind:

- To help individuals who may be candidates for transplant surgery understand the organ donation and transplantation process.
- To ensure that people waiting for donor organs are taking steps to keep as healthy as possible and be ready when that important phone call comes.
- To prepare transplant recipients, and those caring for them, for the recovery process and life after a transplant.
- To offer helpful tips to caregivers who play a vital role in all steps of organ transplantation.
- To encourage organ donation.
- Most important, to let transplant recipients know that they can live long and meaningful lives after transplant surgery.

The book focuses on the most common adult and pediatric organ transplants. Within the chapters, you'll also find information specifically for caregivers and insights from transplant recipients.

It's our hope that our experiences in preparing patients for transplant surgery and caring for them afterward can help you find a transplant center, be prepared for the journey ahead, and ensure a good outcome after transplantation.

1

When a transplant is needed

In 1953, a 22-year-old man named Richard Herrick was discharged from the U.S. Coast Guard with chronic kidney disease, which at the time was an incurable and life-threatening illness. Surgeons had yet to achieve a successful kidney transplant because the transplant recipient's body would inevitably reject the donated organ as genetically different tissue and therefore potentially dangerous.

But Richard proved to be a special case because he had a genetically identical twin who donated one of his kidneys to Richard. Because the tissue of his brother's organ was so like his own, Richard's body accepted the transplant, and he became the first successful kidney transplant recipient. Richard went on to marry his nurse and have two children.

When an organ such as a kidney fails, receiving a new one can be lifesaving. It allows people to live longer, spend more time with the ones they love, travel and pursue hobbies, and build families and fulfilling careers. In the United States alone, since national recording by the Organ Procurement and Transplant Network (OPTN) began in 1988, more than 1 million people have had their lives extended and often significantly improved thanks to organ transplants.

Modern medicine can currently achieve successful transplantation of the following organs:

- Kidney.
- Heart.
- Lung.
- Pancreas.
- Liver.
- Small intestine.

TRANSPLANTS IN ANCIENT HISTORY

Scientists found the first-ever documented case of a skin graft for burns in the Ebers Papyrus, an ancient Egyptian medical record with origins around 1550 B.C. In India, surgeon Sushruta, sometimes referred to as the father of surgery, also delved into skin grafts, dating back to 600 B.C. And one ancient text from 348 A.D. mentions an attempt to replace a patient's cancerous leg with a leg of a recently deceased man. Overall, the idea of transferring body parts between people appears in Roman, Greek, Indian, Chinese and Egyptian legends, with procedures usually performed by gods or healers.

Today, transplant medicine is a rapidly growing field. According to the OPTN, U.S. surgeons performed 48,149 organ transplants in 2024, an increase over the previous year. Since the first successful kidney transplant in 1954, the number of solid organ transplants in the United States now exceeds 1 million, more than any other country in the world. Despite such progress, work remains. The Health Resources and Services Administration estimates that more than 100,000 people are awaiting a transplant and every eight minutes a new person is added to the list.

These vital organs can stop working properly due to several factors, including disease, a congenital defect, or lifestyle factors such as smoking or excessive alcohol consumption.

Eventually — sometimes after years of declining health — the organs can even fail. And when medications and other treatments are no longer effective, an organ transplant may be the only lifesaving option remaining.

BENEFITS AND RISKS OF TRANSPLANT SURGERY

The main benefit of having a transplant is the opportunity to live. For many people, transplant surgery also offers the opportunity to resume a typical life, including work, family activities, travel and hobbies — things that make life enjoyable and worthwhile. Depending on the organ being transplanted, transplant may provide:

- Reduced risk of early death.
- Better quality of life.
- Fewer dietary restrictions.
- Lower lifetime treatment cost.

The goal of organ transplantation is to save lives. And while all transplant recipients must take medication for the rest of their lives, many people are able to resume their usual activities.

Though transplants can extend life, they're not without risks. They are major, invasive surgeries that come with their own potential complications. Recipients must be vigilant about their health and the possibility of rejection after a transplant. Medications taken after transplantation to prevent organ rejection come with their own set of risks and side effects (see Chapter 13).

What's rejection?

All biological cells, whether human or otherwise, are covered with microscopic proteins called antigens that are part of the body's immune system. The immune system is designed to defend the body from anything that's genetically foreign. For example, when germs enter your body, specific antigens on the germs trigger your immune system to produce extra immune cells and protective antibodies to

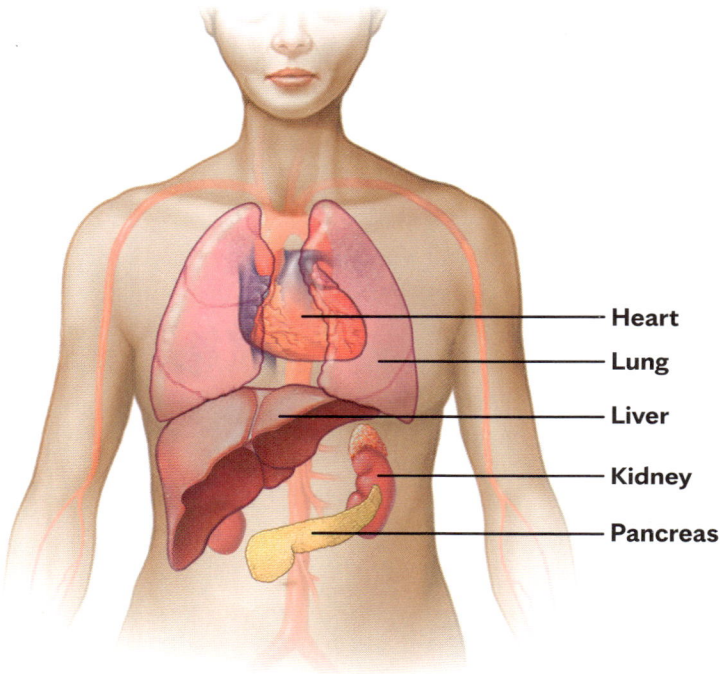

clear out the germs. Your body's cells have their own various antigens, but your immune system recognizes that they belong in your system.

A donor's organ cells have their own antigens as well. When a donor's organ is transplanted into a recipient, the recipient's immune system sees the transplanted tissue as foreign and initiates a response against it. This immune response is referred to as rejection of the transplanted organ. The only time this doesn't happen is when the donor and the recipient are identical twins, as in Richard Herrick's case.

To prevent rejection, recipients of organ transplants must take medications for the remainder of their lives to suppress their immune systems and prevent rejection. Modern antirejection medications, also known as immunosuppressants, are very effective. As long as they are taken as instructed by the medical team, chances of avoiding rejection — and of treating early signs of rejection should they develop — are very good.

Antirejection medications versus immunosuppressants
Perhaps you've seen the terms *antirejection medications* and *immuno-suppressants* used in various materials you've read. And you may have wondered what the difference is between the two. There isn't any. They are two different names that describe the same medications.

Antirejection medicines keep your immune system from attacking healthy cells and tissues by mistake. More specifically, these medicines prevent your immune system from rejecting your new organ. Rejection happens because your immune system knows the transplanted organ is new to your body, and it reacts to it like it would to any intruder. It wants to destroy it.

YOUR TRANSPLANT JOURNEY AT A GLANCE

1. Referral to a transplant center by your healthcare team.
2. Comprehensive evaluation at a transplant center.
3. Acceptance as a transplant candidate and placement on the organ waiting list.
4. If applicable, evaluation of a living donor.
5. Development of a support system and financial strategy.
6. Wait for an organ offer.
7. Transplant surgery at a transplant center.
8. Post-transplant recovery period.
9. Lifelong immunosuppressive therapy.
10. Monitoring by transplant care team.

Because antirejection medicines suppress, which means "hold back," the functioning of your body's immune system, they're also referred to as immunosuppressants. In addition to preventing organ rejection, immunosuppressants are used to treat autoimmune diseases such as rheumatoid arthritis, inflammatory bowel disease and multiple sclerosis.

Antirejection medications are a great discovery that has made it possible for people to live with transplanted organs. However, because these medicines weaken the body's immune system, those who take them are more susceptible to infections and other medical conditions.

KIDNEY TRANSPLANT

A kidney transplant is a surgery to place a healthy kidney from a living or deceased donor into a person whose kidneys are no longer functioning properly.

The kidneys are two bean-shaped organs located on each side of the spine just below the rib cage. Each kidney is about the size of a fist. The kidneys' main function is to filter and remove waste, minerals and fluid from blood by producing urine.

Certain chronic health conditions — including diabetes, high blood pressure, recurring kidney infections and chronic inflammation — as well as some genetic diseases can damage the kidneys and make them gradually lose this filtering ability. In some people, the kidneys may shut down suddenly due to acute kidney injury after a severe illness, complications of surgery, a heart attack or other serious issues. Certain medications also can cause kidney injury.

When kidneys don't function properly, harmful levels of fluid and waste can build up in the body and become life-threatening. Treatment for chronic kidney disease focuses on slowing the progression of kidney damage, usually by controlling the cause.

But sometimes even controlling the cause might not keep kidney damage from worsening. In some cases, chronic kidney disease progresses to end-stage, life-threatening kidney failure, also known as renal failure. End-stage kidney disease occurs when the kidneys lose about 90% of their typical functioning ability.

Common causes of end-stage kidney disease include:

- Type 1 or type 2 diabetes.
- Chronic unmanaged high blood pressure.
- Glomerulonephritis, an inflammation of the kidney's filtering units called glomeruli. It may develop as a complication of another illness, such as an infectious disease or autoimmune condition.
- Interstitial nephritis, an inflammation of the kidney's tubules and surrounding structures. It also often develops as a complication of another health condition.
- Inherited kidney diseases such as polycystic kidney disease.
- Prolonged obstruction of the urinary tract from conditions such as an enlarged prostate, kidney stones and some cancers.

THE KIDNEYS

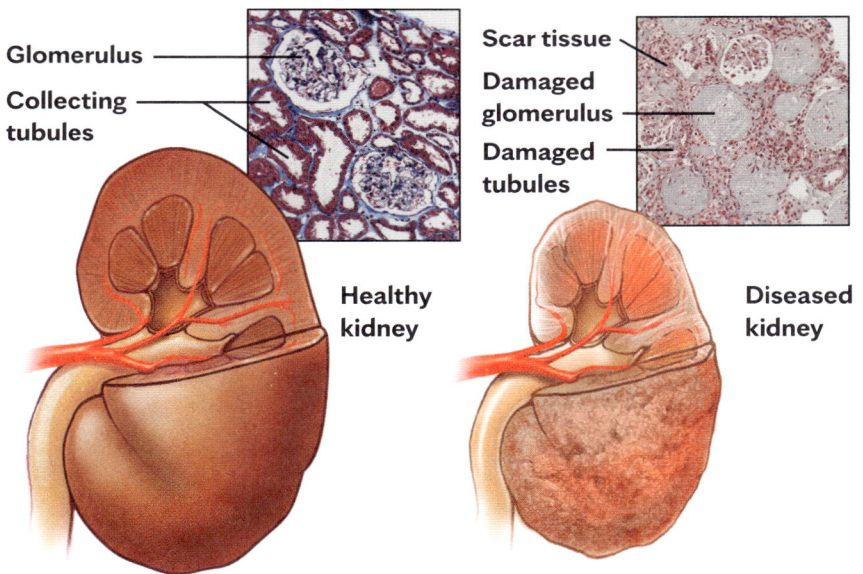

Glomerulus

Collecting tubules

Scar tissue

Damaged glomerulus

Damaged tubules

Healthy kidney

Diseased kidney

A typical kidney has about 1 million filtering units, called glomeruli, that are connected with tiny tubelike structures called tubules. Conditions such as high blood pressure or elevated blood sugar levels take a toll on kidney function by damaging the filtering units and tubules and causing scarring. Unmanaged, these conditions can lead to kidney failure.

STAGES OF KIDNEY DISEASE

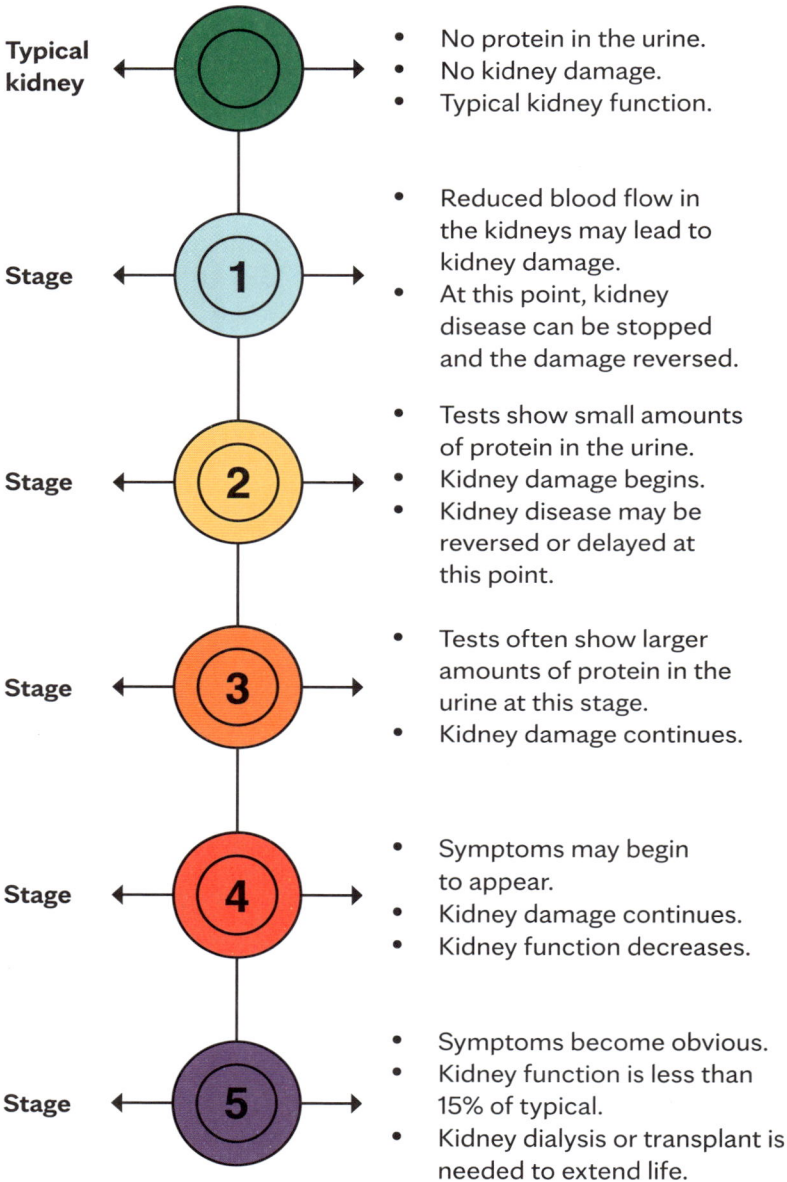

Typical kidney

- No protein in the urine.
- No kidney damage.
- Typical kidney function.

Stage 1

- Reduced blood flow in the kidneys may lead to kidney damage.
- At this point, kidney disease can be stopped and the damage reversed.

Stage 2

- Tests show small amounts of protein in the urine.
- Kidney damage begins.
- Kidney disease may be reversed or delayed at this point.

Stage 3

- Tests often show larger amounts of protein in the urine at this stage.
- Kidney damage continues.

Stage 4

- Symptoms may begin to appear.
- Kidney damage continues.
- Kidney function decreases.

Stage 5

- Symptoms become obvious.
- Kidney function is less than 15% of typical.
- Kidney dialysis or transplant is needed to extend life.

- Vesicoureteral reflux, a condition that causes urine to back up into the kidneys.
- Recurrent kidney infection, also called pyelonephritis.

People who have kidney failure must undergo dialysis. With the help of machines, dialysis does some of the work that the kidneys no longer can do. This includes removing extra fluids and waste products from blood, restoring electrolyte levels and helping control blood pressure. Dialysis has its own list of complications, however, ranging from infections to anemia. A kidney transplant is often the treatment of choice for kidney failure compared with a lifetime of dialysis.

HEART TRANSPLANT

A heart transplant is an operation in which a failing heart is replaced with a healthier donor heart. Heart transplants are used to treat people with end-stage heart failure or other severe heart conditions that don't respond to medication, other therapies or surgery.

When heart failure occurs, the heart can't pump enough blood to meet the body's demand. That doesn't mean that the heart has stopped working completely, but it indicates that the heart isn't working properly. People with end-stage heart failure have difficulty doing everyday physical tasks. The failure tends to worsen over time.

In adults, heart failure can be caused by:

- A weakening of the heart muscle, also called cardiomyopathy.
- Coronary artery disease, which narrows the arteries and increases the risk of heart attack.
- Heart valve disease, in which one or more heart valves don't work properly. This can cause blood to flow in the wrong direction.
- A heart problem you're born with, also known as a congenital heart defect.
- Dangerous recurring irregular heart rhythms, known as ventricular arrhythmias, that are not controlled by other treatments.
- Failure of a previous heart transplant.

While a heart transplant is a major operation, your chance of survival is good with appropriate follow-up care.

Right atrium

Right ventricle

Left atrium

Left ventricle

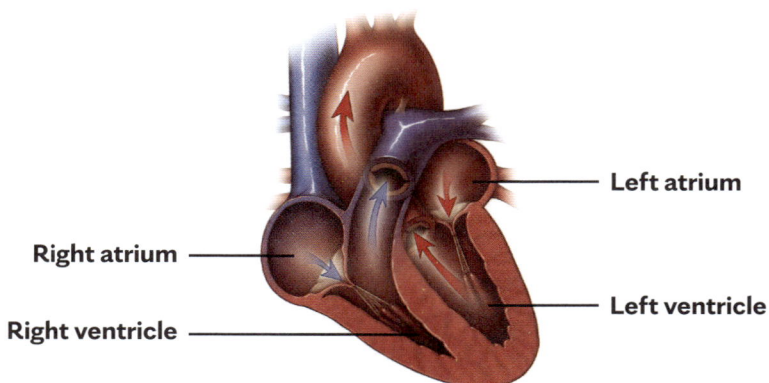

Systolic heart failure

Less blood is pumped out

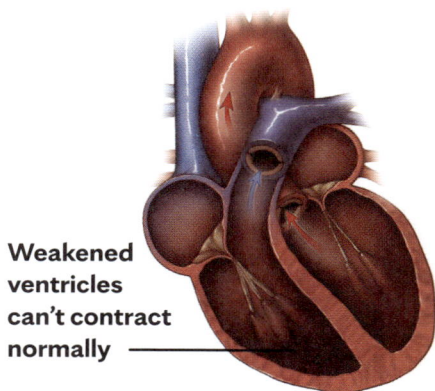

Diastolic heart failure

Less blood enters the ventricle

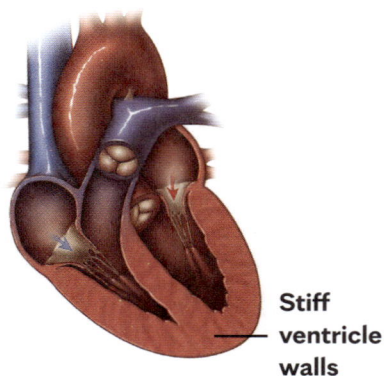

Weakened ventricles can't contract normally

Stiff ventricle walls

The top image shows chambers of the heart. Blood flows into the right side of the heart and from there into the lungs, where it picks up oxygen (blue arrows). Then it flows from the lungs back into the left atrium. From there, it flows into the left ventricle and out to the body (red arrows). Heart failure, as shown in the bottom two images, can result when a weakened, damaged or stiff heart can no longer effectively pump the needed amount of blood. A heart transplant may be an option for treatment.

LIVER TRANSPLANT

A liver transplant is surgery to remove a liver that's no longer function-ing properly and replace it with a healthy liver. The donated liver may come from a deceased donor, or it may be a portion of a healthy liver from a living donor. Receiving a portion of a liver from a living donor is an alternative to waiting for a deceased-donor liver. Living-donor liver transplant is possible because — unlike most organs — the human liver can regenerate and regrow to its typical size shortly after the surgeons remove part of it for transplantation.

Your liver is your largest internal organ, and it performs several critical functions, including:
* Processing nutrients, medications and hormones.
* Producing bile, which helps the body absorb fats, cholesterol and fat-soluble vitamins.
* Making proteins that help the blood clot.
* Removing bacteria and toxins from the blood.
* Preventing infection and regulating immune responses.

THE LIVER

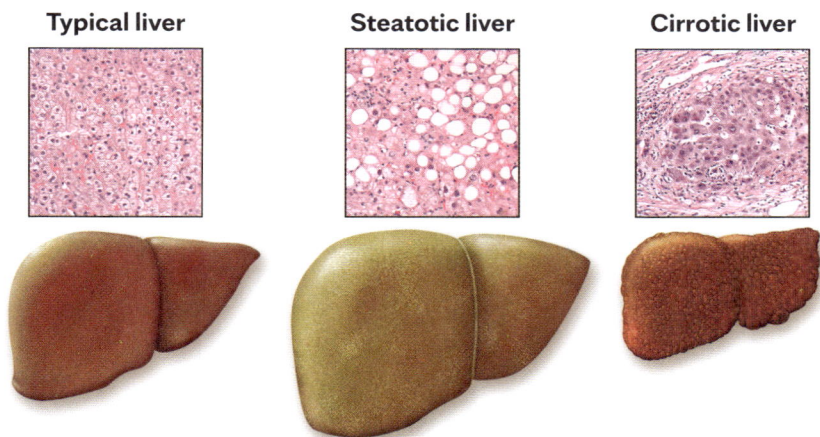

A typical liver (left) shows no sign of scarring. A steatotic liver (middle) is enlarged. A cirrhotic liver (right) shows extensive scarring and shrinkage, which can lead to liver failure.

Liver transplant is an option for people with liver failure who can't be helped by other treatments. Liver failure may happen quickly or over a long period of time.

Liver failure that occurs quickly, in a matter of days to weeks, is called acute liver failure. Acute liver failure is an uncommon condition that may occur as a complication from taking certain medications or due to infections, though in some cases of acute liver failure, the cause is not known.

Chronic liver failure occurs slowly over months and years and may be caused by a variety of conditions. The most common cause of chronic liver failure is scarring of the liver, called cirrhosis. When cirrhosis occurs, scar tissue replaces typical liver tissue, and the liver doesn't function properly.

Cirrhosis is the most frequent reason for a liver transplant. Major causes of cirrhosis leading to liver failure and liver transplant include:

- Alcohol-associated liver disease, which causes damage to the liver due to excessive alcohol consumption.
- Metabolic dysfunction-associated steatotic liver disease, a condition in which fat builds up in the liver, causing inflammation or liver cell damage.
- Hepatitis B and, less commonly, hepatitis C, which are viral diseases that cause liver inflammation.
- Genetic diseases affecting the liver. They include hemochromatosis, which causes excessive iron buildup in the liver, and Wilson's disease, which causes excessive copper buildup in the liver.
- Diseases that affect the tubes that carry bile away from the liver, called the bile ducts. They include primary biliary cirrhosis, primary sclerosing cholangitis and biliary atresia. Biliary atresia is the most common reason for liver transplant among children.

Liver transplant is most often used as a treatment option for people who have significant liver damage due to end-stage chronic liver disease. Liver transplant also may be a treatment option in rare cases of sudden failure of a previously healthy liver.

LUNG TRANSPLANT

A lung transplant replaces a diseased or failing lung with a healthy lung. A lung transplant is typically reserved for people who have tried medications and other treatments for their condition, but it hasn't sufficiently improved.

Having a damaged or diseased lung can make it difficult for the body to get the oxygen it needs to survive. A variety of diseases and conditions can damage the lungs and keep them from functioning effectively. Some of the more common causes include:

- Chronic obstructive pulmonary disease (COPD), including emphysema caused by smoking, pollution or other factors.
- Pulmonary fibrosis, in which lung tissue becomes damaged and scarred.
- Cystic fibrosis, a genetic condition in which sticky, thick mucus builds up in the lungs and other organs of the body.
- Pulmonary hypertension, characterized by high blood pressure in the lungs.

THE LUNGS

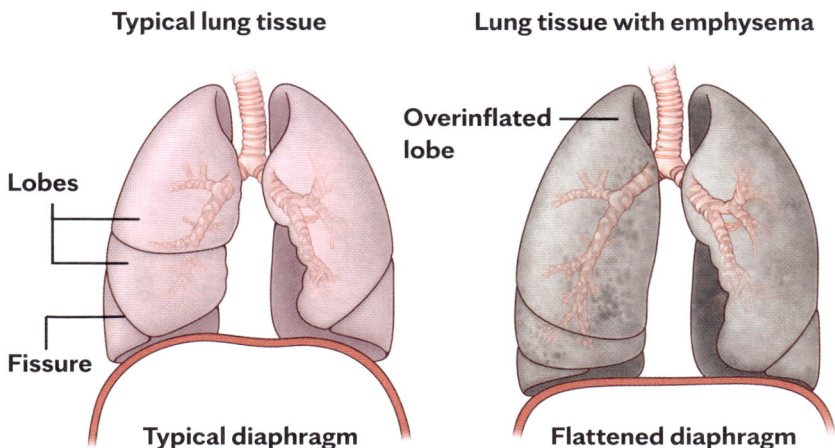

Typical lung tissue

Lung tissue with emphysema

Overinflated lobe

Lobes

Fissure

Typical diaphragm

Flattened diaphragm

Emphysema, a chronic lung disease, is one of a handful of conditions that can lead to lung failure.

Lung damage can often be treated with medication or special breathing devices. But sometimes these measures don't help. For example, lung damage caused by pulmonary fibrosis cannot be repaired. Medicines and therapies can sometimes help slow down the rate of scarring, ease symptoms and improve quality of life, but for some people, the best option is a lung transplant.

If your lung function becomes so poor that it's life-threatening, your healthcare team might suggest a single-lung transplant — receiving one donated lung — or a double-lung transplant — receiving two donated lungs. Sometimes, people with serious heart and lung conditions may need a combined heart-lung transplant.

While a lung transplant is a complex operation that can have complications, it also can greatly improve your health and quality of life.

PANCREAS TRANSPLANT

Pancreas transplant surgery involves the placement of a healthy pancreas into a recipient with diabetes whose pancreas is no longer producing insulin or doesn't produce enough insulin.

The pancreas lies behind the lower part of the stomach. One of its main functions is to make insulin, a hormone that regulates the absorption of blood sugar, also called glucose, into cells. If the pancreas doesn't make enough insulin, blood sugar levels can rise to unhealthy levels, resulting in diabetes.

Most pancreas transplants are performed to treat type 1 diabetes. In type 1 diabetes, the pancreas makes little or no insulin. It most often appears during childhood or adolescence.

A pancreas transplant offers a potential cure for this condition, but it's typically reserved for those with serious complications of diabetes. In some individuals, pancreas transplants also may treat type 2 diabetes. This condition, which is more common in adulthood, occurs when the body's cells become resistant to insulin. A pancreas transplant may be considered for people with any of the following:
- Type 1 diabetes that cannot be managed with standard treatment.
- Frequent insulin reactions.
- Consistent trouble with blood sugar management.
- Severe kidney damage from long-term diabetes.

- Type 2 diabetes associated with both low insulin resistance and low insulin production.

People whose kidneys have been damaged by diabetes may need kidney transplants with a pancreas transplant. There are several different types of pancreas transplants, including:

- **Pancreas transplant alone.** People with diabetes and early or no kidney disease may be candidates for a pancreas transplant alone.
- **Combined kidney-pancreas transplant.** This type of transplant, also called a simultaneous kidney-pancreas transplant, is for people with diabetes who have or are at risk of kidney failure. The goal is to provide a healthy kidney and pancreas that are unlikely to contribute to diabetes-related kidney damage in the future.
- **Pancreas-after-kidney transplant.** For individuals facing a long wait for both a donor kidney and a donor pancreas to become available, a kidney transplant may be recommended first if a living- or deceased-donor kidney becomes available. After recovery from kidney transplant surgery, a pancreas is transplanted once one becomes available.
- **Pancreatic islet cell transplant.** With this type of transplant, insulin-producing cells, called islet cells, taken from a donor's pancreas are injected into a vein that takes blood to the liver. More than one injection of transplanted islet cells may be needed. Islet cell transplantation is being studied for people with serious, progressive complications of type 1 diabetes. Currently, the surgery is only performed as part of a clinical trial approved by the U.S. Food and Drug Administration (FDA).

OTHER AREAS OF TRANSPLANT MEDICINE

The field of transplant medicine is expanding beyond some of the more common organ transplants. Other emerging or less common areas of transplant medicine include the following.

Transplant oncology

A liver transplant may be an option for people with liver cancer who have small tumors that haven't grown into nearby blood vessels,

COMPARING TRANSPLANT CENTERS

One of the most common questions for a transplant team is, "What are the chances of success?" There are statistics for every kind of transplant. But they only tell part of the story. Your chance of a successful transplant or survival depends on many factors. The type of transplant, your overall health and age, the type of donor, and events that occur before, during and after transplant all matter.

You can compare transplant center statistics using an online database maintained by the Scientific Registry of Transplant Recipients (see Additional resources). The database tells you how many transplants a center performs, how the center rates in getting organs to people on waitlists and how long people survive after transplant at the center. You can compare the numbers to national statistics.

You also should check to see whether a transplant center offers other services you might need. These include coordinating support groups, assisting with travel arrangements, helping you find local housing for your recovery period or directing you to organizations that can help with these concerns.

haven't spread outside the liver and can't be surgically removed. Called transplant oncology, this is a potential treatment for people with liver cancer. Recent studies have found that replacing a liver that has cancer with a healthy liver can considerably increase a person's survival time. For some people with hepatocellular carcinoma, the most common type of liver cancer, or in some patients with bile duct cancer, a liver transplant may be the only hope for a cure.

Face and hand transplants
Face and hand transplants are promising new procedures that can restore quality of life for people with disfiguring facial injuries or lost

hands or fingers. In 2016, Mayo Clinic surgeons performed their first near-total face transplant in a 32-year-old Wyoming man. The surgery, which took over 50 hours, involved restoring his nose, upper and lower jaw, palate, teeth, cheeks, facial muscles, and other parts of his face. (To learn more, read *Face in the Mirror: A Surgeon, a Patient, and the Remarkable Story of the First Face Transplant at Mayo Clinic* by Jack El-Hai.) A second successful face transplant was conducted at Mayo Clinic in 2024.

Mayo Clinic surgeons also perform hand transplants, in which they reattach skin, bone, muscles, nerves, tendons and blood vessels.

Small intestine transplant

Small intestine transplant, also known as bowel transplant, involves replacing a small bowel with disease or a shortened small bowel with a

ORGAN TRANSPLANTS AT MAYO CLINIC

Mayo Clinic is the largest integrated transplant provider in the nation. Every year, more than 150 surgeons and physicians perform more than 2,000 solid organ adult and pediatric transplants at Mayo Clinic's campuses in Arizona, Florida and Minnesota.

"Transplant is a highly complex clinical practice that requires a high degree of coordination throughout the patient journey," says C. Burcin Taner, M.D., chair of the Mayo Clinic enterprise Transplant Specialty Council and Mayo Clinic's Transplant Center in Florida. "The growing volume of transplants at Mayo Clinic is the ultimate testament that our patients trust our collective expertise."

Mayo Clinic performed its first organ transplant in 1963. Since then, Mayo scientists and surgeons have remained on the leading edge of transplant medicine, continually improving techniques and expanding technologies. Research activities at Mayo Clinic directly contribute to successful outcomes of organ transplantation nationwide.

bowel from a healthier donor. It can be a lifesaving treatment for short bowel syndrome, in which the small intestine has been damaged or surgically removed. A transplant also may be an option for intestinal failure, in which the bowel can no longer absorb the water and nutrients necessary for sustaining life.

Bone marrow transplant

Bone marrow is the soft material inside bones that produces blood cells the body needs for many functions. A bone marrow transplant is a procedure that infuses healthy blood-forming stem cells into the body to replace bone marrow that's not producing enough healthy blood cells. A bone marrow transplant also is called a stem cell transplant.

You might need a bone marrow transplant if your bone marrow stops working. This type of transplant also is a treatment for cancer that has formed in blood cells, such as leukemia, lymphoma or multiple myeloma.

This book focuses on solid organ transplants. However, some of the information on staying healthy after transplantation, and on medications that may be needed after a transplant, also may be helpful for people having bone marrow transplantation.

FOR CAREGIVERS: YOU ARE THE KEY TO TRANSPLANT SUCCESS

Being a caregiver is a serious commitment and a long-term responsibility. Caregivers must be able to stay with the person receiving the transplant 24 hours a day, seven days a week. An organ transplant is often a life-changing event both for the recipient and the recipient's caregiver.

Research shows that people who have supportive caregivers are more likely to be successful with their transplants. This is because they take their medications regularly, they don't forget to refill their medications, and they attend their appointments on time. They also exercise as they should, eat nutritionally rich foods and avoid foods that may interfere with their transplants.

For someone caring for a person with a serious illness, the possibility of an organ transplant can be exciting but also overwhelming when considering the tasks ahead. If you are a caregiver, you play a vital role in the success of the transplant by providing physical and emotional support before and after the surgery.

In each chapter ahead, you can find special sections for caregivers that contain practical strategies for successfully navigating the transplant journey. For now, consider these basic tips:

Stay organized and have a schedule

Keep a calendar to track appointments, medication schedules and other important events. Maintaining a schedule, whether on paper or digitally, can help you and the person in your care keep track of medical visits, health goals and key milestones.

Communicate with everyone involved

Organ transplant is a complex procedure. You'll likely have many questions at different decision points, as well as various discussions with the person you care for and the medical team. Communicate regularly with everyone involved. Don't hesitate to ask questions or request clarification on issues you don't understand.

Remain patient and positive

Organ transplant is a physically and emotionally challenging journey. The person in your care may experience mood swings or outbursts of frustration, stress or sadness. The person also may have reactions to medications or feel depressed. They may have doubts about the success of a transplant or worry about the surgery and recovery.

You may experience many of the same emotions. Do your best to stay calm, patient and positive to help your loved one. But also remember that it's OK to reach out for help, whether it's from a family member, friend, trusted adviser or mental health professional.

2

Getting evaluated

A NEW HEART FOR A NEW MOM
PROMISE'S STORY

Promise grew up with a congenital heart defect. She was born with transposition of the great arteries, where her heart vessels and her heart weren't correctly configured. This prevented her heart from providing adequate blood flow to the rest of her body. By the time Promise was 24, she had undergone two surgeries to address heart issues. But she was in good health and life was moving forward.

In 2022, she and her husband, Andrew, who serves in the Navy, learned the exciting news that they were going to have a baby.

About six months into her pregnancy, Promise began to struggle. The toll of carrying a growing baby led to complications, including congestive heart failure. "I was fine for the first couple of months, and then the third trimester came, and my body could not handle the fluid shifts," says Promise. "Due to that, I ended up in cardiogenic shock, which is pretty much where your whole body is just shutting down because your heart is no longer [pumping] like it's supposed to."

Promise's son, Paxton, was born 11 weeks early in June. He spent two months in a neonatal intensive care unit. Throughout this time, Promise's health continued to decline due to heart failure. She was in and out of several hospitals as teams tried to determine the best course for her care. Ultimately, Promise and her family made the decision to go to Mayo Clinic.

When Promise arrived at Mayo Clinic, doctors immediately knew that she needed to be transferred to the intensive care unit (ICU), where temporary pumps and medication helped keep her alive until her care team could determine if she was a candidate for a transplant and could survive one. Two days later, she was added to the heart transplant list.

"It became very evident that in order to optimize her care, we needed to know what we were getting into, how her heart position was actually related to her chest wall, and how her vessels were within her chest," says Parag C. Patel, M.D., a Mayo Clinic transplant cardiologist. "So, we reached out to our 3D printing team and asked them to reconstruct a model of Promise's heart."

The 3D renderings helped the team to quickly establish a game plan. The surgeons were able to reference the model in the operating room even as they performed her procedure. "Because of the collaborative approach and high level of communication with each of the members of our multidisciplinary team, we were able to take separate pieces of technology and cater our therapies and tailor it for Promise," says Dr. Patel.

Promise received her new heart in September 2022. She has since celebrated many milestones, including her son's first birthday, her 25th birthday and her second transplant anniversary.

"Being on that operating room table as a new mom, as a wife, a daughter, I think the biggest thought was I had to pull through this surgery for my son — if not for myself, my husband, my mom and my brother — for my son. My son needed me," says Promise.

If you're living with severe heart failure, kidney failure or another illness that can cause organ decline, you and your healthcare team may determine that a transplant is the best treatment option.

Because so many factors play a role in a successful organ transplant, you must first undergo a comprehensive evaluation to make sure that you're a good candidate for transplantation. A transplant candidate must be healthy enough to undergo the complex procedure and the extended recovery involved. The candidate also must be prepared to live with a transplant, which includes taking medications daily for life to prevent rejection of the new organ.

Life after transplant also involves other lifestyle changes, such as exercising and eating a healthy diet, which sometimes includes avoiding certain foods. In addition, transplant candidates must have at least one person to provide support for them during evaluation and transplant recovery.

Another key factor is that your insurance company must approve your evaluation for transplant as well as approve the procedure before you can be placed on a waiting list. See Chapter 3 for more information on the financial aspects of transplant surgery.

MEETING WITH YOUR TRANSPLANT CARE TEAM

If your healthcare team determines that you need a transplant, you'll be referred to a transplant program within a medical center. Each transplant program uses certain criteria to decide whether to accept a person as a transplant candidate.

At the transplant program, you'll meet with a transplant care team. The care team will review your medical history, ask you questions and guide you through a series of medical tests. Different types of transplants may require different tests.

The transplant care team typically includes a transplant coordinator, social worker, transplant doctor, surgeon, pharmacist and other specialists, such as dietitians and financial coordinators. The team also may include doctors trained in specialty areas such as anesthesia, imaging, psychology and specific diseases — heart, lung, blood, kidney, liver and infectious diseases.

During a transplant evaluation, you'll likely meet with a:

- **Clinical transplant coordinator.** This is a nurse with specialized transplant training who will help you understand the evaluation process, the organ waiting list, and what you need to do before and after transplant. The clinical transplant coordinator will answer your questions and help you become fully informed about the transplant process. The coordinator also will coordinate the care you receive while you are waiting for your transplant, as well as the care you receive after your transplant.

- **Transplant social worker.** This individual will talk with you about your ability to cope with the stress of the transplant and your ability to follow a treatment plan. The social worker also can help you identify your support network and develop a plan for who will take care of you and where you will stay after the surgery.
- **Transplant financial coordinator.** The role of the financial coordinator is to help you understand the costs associated with your transplant and the lifelong medications you'll need to take after the transplant. A financial coordinator may also work with you to understand your insurance coverage. Some costs may not be covered by insurance. Both the financial coordinator and the social worker can help identify other resources for which you may be eligible, to help fill any gaps in your insurance coverage.
- **Transplant registered dietitian.** A registered dietitian will review your nutritional needs, address any problem areas and provide nutritional education about foods that are safe before and after transplant.
- **Transplant pharmacist.** A pharmacist helps make sure you understand how to take your medications correctly. The transplant pharmacist also reviews your current medications to make sure there are no interactions with the medications prescribed after transplant.

This assessment may be done in person, by phone or by looking at your medical record. If you're being evaluated for a kidney or liver transplant, your medical team also will likely discuss a living-donor option with you. You can read more about deceased versus living donors on pages 78-79.

Medical history and general health exam

The transplant care team will ask you about any illnesses, previous surgeries and treatments you've had. You'll be checked for cancer;

IS AGE A FACTOR?

When determining whether someone should receive a transplant, many transplant teams place more significance on an adult's overall health — the person's physiological age — than just on chronological age.

For example, frailty — a limited capacity to respond to stress or bounce back from injury or surgery — seems to be an important factor, as it has been linked with health problems after transplantation, including an increased risk of premature death.

Older adults undergoing a transplant may have more hurdles, including:

- **Coexisting health needs.** It's common for older adults to take several medications, some of which could potentially interact with immune system suppression medicines that are necessary after transplant surgery to prevent organ rejection. It's also common for older adults to have chronic illnesses that a transplant can't fix, making a transplant less likely to be helpful.
- **Side effects of therapy after transplant surgery.** Immune system suppression medicines, known as antirejection medicines or immunosuppressants, can aggravate existing medical conditions, such as tremor, diabetes, kidney failure and high blood pressure.

On the positive side, immune systems naturally weaken with age. This might work to the advantage of older organ recipients by lowering their chances of acute organ rejection.

Overall, Mayo Clinic experts say that when older transplant candidates are carefully screened and selected, they can experience excellent results.

infections; diseases of the liver, lung and heart; and other conditions that might impair recovery after a transplant.

You'll need to keep your dental care current to make sure you don't have any active cavities, infections or gum disease. These issues can cause problems after transplant.

Psychosocial evaluation

You and your caregiver likely will meet with a social worker to discuss your care before and after transplant surgery. This meeting is to make sure you're emotionally prepared for surgery, recovery and living with a new organ. Many aspects of the transplant journey can be stressful. A psychosocial evaluation aims to ensure that you have all the right tools and resources to cope with the physical and emotional aspects of this process. (See additional information for caregivers later in this chapter.)

Additionally, your social worker or financial coordinator will explain to you the financial aspects of transplant surgery, from medications to lodging. You can read more about the financial aspects of organ transplantation in Chapter 3.

A social worker may ask you various questions, including about your health history, your employment situation and your feelings about transplant. The social worker will discuss the importance of having a caregiver during all stages of organ transplant — evaluation, waitlist, surgery and recovery. It's important for you to understand the risks and benefits of having a transplant and to address any concerns you might have.

COMPATIBILITY TESTS

A transplant evaluation also includes gathering biological information to help with finding a suitable donor. Most transplant recipients receive an organ from someone who has at least some genetic differences, even if the donor and recipient are closely related. The exception is when the donor and the recipient are identical twins.

Immunologic blood and tissue matching is one of many factors that play a role in determining compatibility of a donor to a recipient. ABO blood type compatibility and the avoidance of preexisting tissue antibodies are crucial for nearly all solid organ transplants.

Sometimes, the transplant team may recommend a special treatment protocol to allow you to receive a transplant from an ABO-incompatible donor. And some organs, such as the liver, seem to be less sensitive to preexisting antibodies. Your transplant team will screen for factors specific to each type of solid organ transplant.

Whether you're receiving an organ from a living donor or a deceased donor, there are systems and best practices in place to ensure the match is compatible.

Blood type

The first compatibility criterion is your blood type. There are four blood types: A, B, AB and O. Some blood types are compatible with each other; others aren't. For example, blood type O from a donor can go to any recipient, but a blood type O recipient can only receive blood from an O (or A2) donor. Blood from an AB donor can only go to an AB recipient, but an AB recipient is compatible with all blood types.

The positive or negative sign associated with blood type, for example, O+ or O-, is related to the presence of a marker on blood cells called the Rh factor. This factor is important for blood transfusion, but it's not something that's important for organ transplantation.

There's also a rare subtype of blood type A, known as subtype A2. Donors with this subtype may be eligible to donate to individuals that people with blood type A normally aren't able to. If your blood type is A, your transplant center can determine if you have the rare subtype.

When you're being evaluated for a transplant, your transplant care team will note your blood type. The team will use this information to find a compatible donor for you. This information is entered into the national system for matching deceased donors to recipients, which is designed to ensure that organ recipients receive a compatible donor organ. There also are rules to try to ensure fairness for waiting recipients of all blood types.

Tissue type

The second compatibility criterion is your tissue type, which you inherit from your parents. Your tissue type is marked by a set of molecules called human leukocyte antigens. This is often abbreviated

BLOOD TYPE MATCHING

If your blood type is:	You can receive an organ from:
Type O	Type O
Type A	Type A or O
Type B	Type B or O
Type AB	Type AB, A, B, or O

to HLA. The HLA test checks for six common antigens that occur in the general population. If you have an identical twin, you share all the same tissue markers. But with most people, you share only some or none with others.

It's not necessary to have a full match, however. Most transplants occur through deceased donors and most are not well matched. A less closely matched donor also can be used. Even when there are no HLA matches — 6 out of 6 mismatches — a transplant may still be successful. The long-term risk of rejection is higher. But the risk can be managed with close monitoring and appropriate use of antirejection medication.

Around 30% of people waiting for a transplant have been exposed, also called sensitized, to other people's HLAs. This means the exposed person's immune system may have developed antibodies against the other HLAs, although this doesn't always happen. Exposure might have happened during a prior transplant, blood transfusion or pregnancy, for example.

Your transplant center will screen your blood sample for any anti-HLA antibodies, as well as their relative amount and strength. Knowing that you have pre-formed antibodies against certain HLAs can help in identifying the best donor match for you. Screening helps you avoid getting an organ that your body is already primed to reject.

Or in cases where a match is still possible, it can impact how much antirejection medication you need to take after transplant. Screening for anti-HLA antibodies is conducted regularly while you're on the waiting list.

Crossmatch

When a donor becomes available — either living or deceased — a third matching test, called a crossmatch test, is done. This test may be performed by way of computer analysis, or it may involve mixing a small sample of your blood with the donor's blood in the lab. The test determines whether anti-HLA antibodies in your blood will likely react against antigens in the donor's blood.

A negative crossmatch means you're compatible and your body isn't as likely to reject the donor organ. Even with a positive crossmatch, a transplant is still possible but requires more medical treatment before and after the transplant to reduce the risk of your antibodies reacting to the donor organ.

ORGAN-SPECIFIC TESTS

Depending on the type of transplant you need, your transplant care team also will use organ-specific tests in your evaluation. Each type of transplant has its own evaluation process to best assess the urgency of the situation and determine the best available treatment options.

In the pages that follow in this chapter, you will read about policies currently in place to guide deceased-donor organ allocation, meaning the factors that are considered to determine the order of which patient will be offered which donor organ. It's important to know that this system continues to be carefully assessed by the Organ Procurement and Transplantation Network (OPTN). Over time updates are made to optimize the system.

Kidney transplant

Kidney failure can have different causes. In the United States, the leading causes of kidney disease include complications related to diabetes and high blood pressure. High levels of blood sugar damage

U.S. TRANSPLANT SYSTEM AT A GLANCE

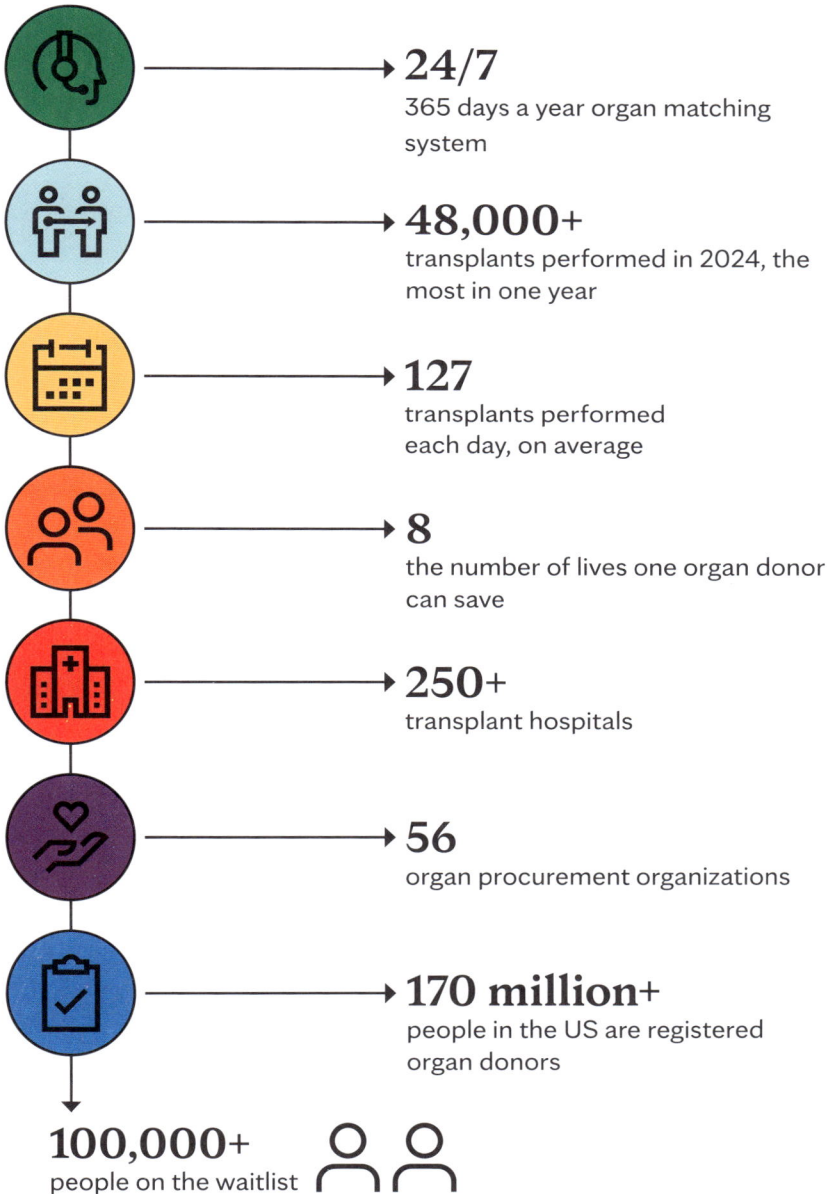

24/7
365 days a year organ matching system

48,000+
transplants performed in 2024, the most in one year

127
transplants performed each day, on average

8
the number of lives one organ donor can save

250+
transplant hospitals

56
organ procurement organizations

170 million+
people in the US are registered organ donors

100,000+
people on the waitlist

Source: United Network for Organ Sharing (UNOS)

A MORE EQUITABLE NEEDS ASSESSMENT

To estimate how well a kidney functions, healthcare teams use a count called eGFR, which stands for estimated glomerular filtration rate. The eGFR shows how well the kidneys filter out a waste compound from blood called creatinine. Creatinine is a byproduct of muscle metabolism, so a person with a larger muscle mass produces higher amounts of creatinine.

A poorly devised historical formula that was widely used in medicine made race a factor in eGFR calculations. It assumed that Black people always have higher muscle mass than do people of other races. Based on the assumption, the formula was adjusted in such a way that it reported a higher amount of kidney function in Black people, even when the function was actually worse.

In 2021, a correction to the kidney function assessment in Black Americans led to more Black people being placed on the kidney transplant list. Until then, healthcare teams used a standard formula to assess kidney function. That formula included an adjustment for Black individuals.

the blood vessels in the kidneys over time, so they no longer work well. Many people who have diabetes also have high blood pressure, which can damage the kidneys further. High blood pressure without diabetes also can cause kidney damage and kidney failure.

About 1 in 3 adults with diabetes has kidney disease, also called diabetic nephropathy. There are many other causes of kidney disease, including some conditions that people are born with. Out of about 100,000 people on the transplant waitlist, approximately 88,000 are waiting for a kidney.

If you're being evaluated for a kidney transplant, you'll undergo comprehensive testing to assess your health and determine the stage of kidney failure. People are eligible to receive kidney transplant once kidney function has decreased to below a specific level — glomerular

"The Black race was used as a variable to calculate eGRF with the assumption that there's more muscle mass in African American people," says Carrie C. Jadlowiec, M.D., a transplant surgeon. "And by adding more muscle mass, the equation was adjusted so that it would show a higher eGFR, thereby potentially delaying the recognition of kidney disease and referral to transplant."

The race-based calculation often delayed the diagnosis of kidney failure as well as the eligibility for a transplant. Consequently, many Black Americans who had improperly calculated and artificially high eGFRs had to wait longer to be referred for transplant evaluations. Many also waited longer to be placed on the transplant waitlist, because their high eGFRs made them appear less critically ill. When the calculation process was corrected in 2021, many Black Americans awaiting a transplant were given additional priority on the waiting list to account for this.

filtration rate (GFR) of 20 milliliters per minute or lower — even if they haven't yet started on dialysis treatment.

There are two additional scores that are unique to kidney transplant. The estimated post-transplant survival (EPTS) score is calculated based on your age, whether you have diabetes, whether you're on dialysis, and how long you have been on dialysis. The EPTS score ranges from 0 to 100 and represents a percentage of how long you may benefit from a kidney transplant compared with others in the registry pool. This score is used to help ensure that recipients receive deceased-donor kidneys with similar life expectancies.

For example, if your EPTS score is close to 0, you'll likely live a long time with the new kidney. If your EPTS score is 10, you'll live with a new kidney longer than 90% of other people. If your EPTS score is close to 100, a new kidney may provide less benefit in terms of longevity.

The scoring process for donor kidneys is similar. It's called a kidney donor profile index (KDPI). It also ranges from 0 to 100. A kidney with a KDPI closer to 0 is expected to function longer than most other kidneys donated by deceased donors. A kidney with a KDPI of 90 may perform well after transplantation but may not last as long as most other kidneys.

OPTN, which manages the national organ transplant system, currently uses the EPTS and KDPI scores to find the right combination between recipients and donors. If your EPTS score is 20 or lower, you'll likely live with a new kidney for a long time. The national allocation system will try to offer you a kidney with a KDPI of 20 or lower.

Whether you receive a kidney from a deceased donor versus a living donor is also a factor in how long the kidney will last. On average, a kidney received from a deceased donor lasts 8 to 12 years. A kidney gifted by a living donor lasts about 15 to 20 years. And some kidneys may last even longer. An additional benefit of living-donor kidney transplant is that it allows recipients to spend less time waiting for a transplant and allows the surgery to be planned for a time when the recipient's medical condition is improved through medication and lifestyle changes.

Heart transplant
People referred for a heart transplant evaluation typically fall within two categories: those who are hospitalized due to the severity of their heart failure and those who aren't in a hospital.

People who are hospitalized typically have a life-threatening illness. Their hearts may have stopped beating. Or they have had a heart attack or another severe injury that has damaged the heart beyond repair. These people are evaluated immediately in a hospital and offered transplants as soon as possible.

People who are still living at home undergo most of the evaluation assessment without being admitted to the hospital. They're usually not critically ill, but their heart health is declining to the point that they'll need a transplant in the near future.

Individuals undergoing heart transplant evaluation generally start with two important tests.

- **Cardiopulmonary stress test.** With this test, an individual walks on a treadmill while breathing into a machine that determines and displays the person's vitals, such as blood pressure.
- **Heart catheterization procedure.** In this procedure, a cardiologist threads a wire with a camera into different parts of the heart to assess how well it's working.

These tests help your medical team determine whether you need a transplant and how soon. If test results indicate you need a transplant, you'll be placed on the national transplant waitlist. The transplant care team will run another round of tests to see what needs to be done to best prepare you for the transplant procedure.

Currently, heart transplant candidates are grouped into categories 1 to 6 according to the severity of their medical conditions, with status 1 being the most urgent. Having a heart that may fail in the near future is ranked more urgent than a heart condition that can be managed by medications.

Criteria for a successful donor match include blood type, HLAs and heart size that's compatible with the transplant candidate. The distance between the donor hospital and recipient hospital also needs to be taken into account.

Lung transplant

Evaluation for a lung transplant includes tests such as a chest X-ray and CT scan and pulmonary function tests. Your transplant care team calculates what's known as your individualized lung Composite Allocation Score (CAS).

The CAS score takes into account your medical condition, age, blood type, how quickly you can get to the transplant center, and other aspects, such as whether you donated an organ in the past.

Each of these factors carries a certain number of points that are added together to a maximum score of 100. Half of the CAS score — up to 50 points — comes from the urgency of the individual's medical condition and the likelihood that the transplant procedure will prolong life.

Someone with a higher number of CAS points more urgently needs a new lung; however, time spent on the waiting list is also a factor. The

A VISIT WITH MAYO CLINIC TRANSPLANT CARDIOLOGIST PARAG C. PATEL, M.D.

When we see patients for a transplant evaluation, we assess them to see if they need a transplant. People who are already in the hospital with heart conditions are usually very sick. These patients won't live long without a transplant, so we evaluate them immediately. We keep them in the hospital, and we get them a transplant quickly.

Patients who aren't hospitalized are typically referred to us by their cardiologists or internal medicine physicians for several reasons. For example, their blood pressure may be too low because the medication isn't working. Or they've come to the hospital a few times because their hearts are too weak. Or they can't do any standard activities, meaning they can't walk a flight of stairs or take a shower without getting short of breath. It also could be that they have dangerously irregular heartbeats. We evaluate them to determine whether they need a transplant.

Not everyone needs a transplant. Sometimes heart health can be improved by adjusting medications or by making lifestyle changes, such as quitting smoking. Even though I'm a transplant physician, if I can avoid transplant and get the patient's heart to work better, that's always best. Mainly because you have to weigh the risks and benefits of transplantation versus other treatment options.

For some people, it may be too early for a transplant. They may have weak hearts, but they could be fine without a transplant for

longer you've been waiting, the more weighted this factor becomes in finding you a match. The CAS score also includes an efficiency component to try to optimize transplant outcomes.

Liver transplant

People are referred for a liver transplant evaluation because they have either acute or chronic liver failure. Chronic liver failure is the most common reason for liver transplant. Chronic liver failure, also called several years. For these people, we try to optimize their medications and lifestyle to make them stronger and healthier. For example, if people are drinking alcohol or smoking, we work with them to help them change their habits and improve their exercise routine.

If we determine that a patient has less than two years to live without the transplant, then the benefits outweigh the risks. In this case, we put them on the transplant list. We'll also assess how critically they need a transplant. If they need an artificial pump to keep their heart going, they'll be higher up on the list. If they need medication through an IV to keep their heart pumping, they'll be in the middle. And if their heart pumping function can be managed with medications, they'll go farther down the list.

At that point, we'll run another round of tests, which are transplant specific. We'll look at our transplant patients from head to toe. We'll make sure they don't have any other health conditions that may interfere with the transplant. If they do, we'll treat the conditions to optimize their health as much as possible. A lot of people do well with heart transplants. The national average for a heart transplant is about 90% survival for the first year. And the average survival total is about 15 years. So transplants extend and improve lives for many people.

cirrhosis, can be caused by different diseases, such as hepatitis infection, chronic excessive alcohol use and steatotic liver disease, formerly known as fatty liver disease. Acute liver failure is a rare condition most commonly caused by an overdose of acetaminophen (Tylenol, others). Use of some supplements and prescription medications also can lead to acute liver failure. And sometimes the cause can't be identified.

People who develop acute liver failure have a very short window of time to receive a liver transplant, usually only a few days. That's because there are no stopgap measures. While kidney failure can be managed with dialysis and heart failure with various devices, at this time there is no machine that can do what the liver does. This is because the liver performs so many different functions, including flushing toxins and bacteria from the bloodstream, making bile to help digest food, and generating proteins to make blood clot.

People with acute liver failure also can recover without a transplant if the liver manages to regenerate itself. Your transplant care team will use specific metrics to evaluate how critically you need a liver transplant.

Evaluation for a liver transplant involves specific blood tests to help your care team calculate your Model for End-Stage Liver Disease (MELD) score. Your MELD score is based on the following measurements:

- Internal normalized ratio (INR) is a number that indicates how well your blood is able to clot.

OBESITY AND LIVER TRANSPLANT SUCCESS

The expanding obesity epidemic in the U.S. has led to a rise in metabolic dysfunction-associated steatotic liver disease, formerly known as nonalcoholic fatty liver disease, which is a leading indication for liver transplant. However, because obesity is a risk factor for serious complications after transplant surgery, many people who would otherwise benefit from transplant don't become candidates for this type of treatment. In other people, a transplant is performed, but the obesity is ignored, leading to poor long-term outcomes.

Julie K. Heimbach, M.D., is the director of the Transplant Center at Mayo Clinic's campus in Rochester, Minnesota. Dr. Heimbach and her colleagues conceived an idea to combine a liver transplant and a weight-loss procedure called sleeve gastrectomy into a single surgery.

- Creatinine level is a measure of the waste product filtered out of the body by your kidney and an indicator of how well your kidneys are working.
- Bilirubin level is an indicator of how well your liver is clearing a substance called bile, which is needed for digestion.
- Serum sodium level is an indicator of how well your body is regulating its fluid balance.
- Recipient sex is the sex assigned at birth, male or female.

The MELD score ranges from 6 to 40. The higher the number, the more urgent the need for a transplant. The MELD score helps predict of the risk of dying of liver failure. The score can be recalculated whenever a patient has a change in health condition.

If an individual has a low score and symptoms are well controlled, then a transplant may be delayed. If symptoms aren't well controlled but the person has a low MELD score, then a living-donor

To investigate its efficacy, the team collected years of follow-up data for dozens of patients who underwent the tandem procedure. They found the approach to be safe and effective in the long term. Compared with people with obesity who underwent liver transplant alone, those who had the double procedure enjoyed better long-term outcomes for weight loss, blood pressure, insulin resistance and fatty liver. They also were less likely to need blood pressure and cholesterol medications.

The double surgery is currently offered at only a handful of hospitals, but its practice is growing. "This procedure can dramatically transform the future for patients who had no other treatment options," Dr. Heimbach says. "Its synergy gives a new freedom to patients who've struggled with obesity their whole lives."

liver transplant also may be considered. An individual with a high MELD score is more likely to get a transplant from a deceased donor. See pages 78-79 for more information on deceased versus living donors.

Some conditions, such as hepatocellular cancer, require a timely transplant to prevent the cancer from enlarging or spreading out of the liver. Even though many of these patients may have lower calculated MELD scores, the increased risk is taken into consideration. These individuals may receive an additional MELD score to prioritize them for a timely transplant.

Because your health may change while you're waiting for a liver transplant, you may need to repeat evaluation tests. Candidates with MELD scores between 6 and 10 need new tests about once a year. Candidates with high MELD scores may need to test as often as once a week.

Pancreas transplant and combined kidney-pancreas transplant

Most pancreas transplants are done to treat type 1 diabetes. Type 1 diabetes is a condition that happens when the pancreas makes little or no insulin. It was once known as juvenile diabetes or insulin-dependent diabetes.

If you have type 1 diabetes and are at risk of kidney failure or you develop a condition called hypoglycemia unawareness, your transplant care team may determine that you need a combined kidney and pancreas transplant. Hypoglycemia unawareness is a condition in which you experience reduced warning symptoms of low blood sugar.

People who receive a pancreas transplant no longer need insulin injections, so transplanting a pancreas and a kidney together treats both the diabetes and the kidney failure. Sometimes this approach can work for people with type 2 diabetes too. Type 2 diabetes happens when the body is not able to use insulin correctly and sugar builds up in the blood. Type 2 diabetes was once called adult-onset diabetes.

If you're being evaluated for a pancreas transplant or a kidney-pancreas transplant, you'll undergo a comprehensive battery of tests. These include checking your levels of insulin and blood sugar to

OTHER MULTIORGAN TRANSPLANTS

In some situations, the best treatment option is to replace multiple organs at once. In addition to a combined kidney-pancreas transplant, multiorgan transplants include the following:

- **Heart-kidney transplant.** This procedure may be an option for some people who have both heart and kidney failure. There are specific criteria to determine who is eligible for this combined transplant.
- **Heart-liver transplant.** This procedure may be an option for people with certain heart and liver conditions.
- **Heart-lung transplant.** Some people with severe lung and heart diseases need a heart transplant and a lung transplant together.
- **Liver-kidney transplant.** This procedure may be an option for certain patients with conditions that affect both the liver and the kidneys. There are specific criteria to determine who is eligible for this type of transplant.

understand how well your pancreas is working. If your transplant care team determines that you're a candidate for a pancreas transplant or a combined kidney-pancreas transplant, you may be placed on the waiting list.

The pancreas allocation score is based on a core set of parameters. They include meeting the medical criteria for a transplant, whether you're waiting for a pancreas or a combined kidney-pancreas, the distance between the donor and your transplant hospital, and how long you've been on the waiting list.

FOR CAREGIVERS: UNDERSTANDING THE EXPECTATIONS
Caring for a transplant patient is a full-time job that will last at least several weeks, if not months, depending on the type of transplant. For

example, recovery from heart, lung and liver transplant surgery often takes longer than recovery from a kidney transplant. You'll need to be the transplant recipient's constant companion for 24 hours a day, seven days a week, for the full recovery period.

During that time, you most likely won't be able to work, especially if you need to travel to the transplant center or temporarily relocate to be near one. In some cases, people are able to work remotely. But in your caregiving role, you'll likely have a full schedule of appointments to attend, which can limit work plans. You may need to ask your employer for a family leave of absence. A social worker can often help with that process and may help you draft a

CAREGIVER CHECKLIST AT A GLANCE

As a caregiver, you must be:
- [ ] At least 18 years old.
- [ ] Able to drive or have a transportation plan.
- [ ] Able to accompany the person in your care to all tests and appointments during the transplant evaluation stage.
- [ ] Able to take off work for the duration of surgery and recovery, which could range from several weeks to several months.
- [ ] Able to travel to the transplant center with the person in your care at a moment's notice.
- [ ] With the transplant recipient 24 hours a day, seven days a week, for the duration of surgery and recovery, which could be several months.
- [ ] Able to accompany the person in your care to all appointments and procedures during the recovery process and pick up the person's medications from the pharmacy.
- [ ] Able to help the person in your care follow the post-transplant medication regimen.
- [ ] Able to take care of yourself, both physically and mentally, throughout the journey.

letter to your employer explaining why your constant presence is required.

Caregiver requirements vary between different centers, but there are several set rules. You must be 18 or older and able to drive the person in your care to appointments and procedures. If you're temporarily relocating, you may need to rent a car. If you're not able to drive, you'll need a comprehensive transportation plan. This might include a combination of hotel shuttle services, public transportation and ride-sharing. Your social worker can help you create a transportation plan.

As a caregiver, you'll be expected to attend the transplant evaluation appointments with the person in your care. Make sure that you understand the transplant process and accompanying requirements. You also may need to help the person in your care understand what lies ahead. Often people referred for a transplant have poor health, so they may be fatigued or have trouble focusing. You also may need to help fill out forms and keep track of appointments.

If you have young children, it might be best to arrange for someone to provide full-time care for them, including meals, transportation to and from child care or school, and bedtime routines. Even if you live close to the transplant hospital and your loved one will be recovering at home, you'll need to stay with your loved one.

Additionally, some transplant centers, including Mayo Clinic, require that you have a backup caregiver, in case anything unexpected happens. Your social worker can help guide you through these preparations. It also may be possible to have the backup caregiver and the primary caregiver work together as a team. But it's essential to agree on a support plan in advance.

3

Deciphering the finances

Part of preparing for a transplant means fully understanding the planning, effort and expenses involved. Many arrangements need to be made ahead of time, such as lodging, transportation, medication, insurance and payment. Understanding what's involved can help you with decisions as you prepare to make the necessary commitments, including financial and other responsibilities. It's important to understand what your insurance will cover, what you're responsible for and any extra expenses you may need to plan for.

If you're employed, check to see if your employer provides disability benefits. Some employers provide short- and long-term disability, which covers some of your salary when you can't work.

The cost of having a transplant is dependent on multiple factors, including insurance coverage. To help you understand and plan for the financial aspects of transplant surgery, a transplant care team typically includes a social worker or financial coordinator or both. These people also can help you explore options to fund your operation, including fundraising and seeking help from nonprofits and patient advocate organizations.

UNDERSTANDING INSURANCE COVERAGE

While you go through your transplant evaluation, a member of the transplant care team or a representative from the medical center's financial office may be assigned to your case to work with your insurance provider on the initial preauthorization for the procedure. This person likely will review your insurance benefits and coverage with you and answer financial questions.

The process can differ from one transplant center to another. But no matter the center you're at, it's necessary to ensure that your insurance company will cover your transplant procedure at that specific medical facility.

Different types of health insurance have different transplant coverage policies.

Private insurance

Private insurance plans, also called commercial insurance plans, cover transplant costs, but their terms and benefits vary. Be prepared to pay for some of the expenses, such as deductibles or copayments, as well as any procedures that your plan doesn't cover. It's also important to know whether your plan covers in-network transplant centers only or whether it offers at least some coverage for out-of-network centers.

Medicare

Medicare is a federal insurance plan for hospital and medical expenses, primarily for older adults, people with disabilities, and people with end-stage kidney disease. Medicare usually covers 80% of transplant expenses, as long as the transplant surgery is performed at a Medicare-approved transplant center. There are some expenses Medicare doesn't cover, such as transportation.

Another variable is whether you have a Medigap policy, a type of health insurance policy sold by private companies that helps cover the out-of-pocket costs not paid by Original Medicare. Medicare Advantage, also known as Part C, is an alternative to Original Medicare, managed by private companies. If you have Medicare Advantage, you can't have a Medigap policy.

Since the options are complex and the implications wide-ranging, you might want to speak with an independent insurance agent in your area. If you're on Medicare, inquire about the free healthcare counseling program Medicare offers to determine what options best fit your situation. See the Additional resources section at the end of this book for more information on Medicare transplant coverage and plans.

Questions to ask

Regardless of the type of coverage you have, clarifying the following questions with your insurance company before you embark on your transplant journey can be extremely helpful.

- Is my transplant center in-network? Is it a Medicare-approved center? An in-network center or a Medicare-approved center is likely to have lower out-of-pocket costs.
- What deductibles will I have to pay?
- What are my co-payments for doctor visits, lab tests, hospital stays and medicines? To get Medicare drug coverage, you must join a Medicare drug plan.
- Do I have prescription coverage, and if so, who is my insurance carrier for prescriptions? You'll want to call the prescription carrier and ask about your medication coverage.
- Does my plan require preauthorization for certain medical procedures? How long does it usually take to obtain preauthorization?
- Does my plan cover transportation and lodging expenses for me and my caregiver? Some Medicare plans don't cover travel and lodging expenses.
- Does my plan have a lifetime maximum or "cap" for transplant services? For travel and lodging expenses? And are there any other caps I should know about?
- Does my policy cover living donor, deceased donor and procurement expenses?
- Is there a waiting period for coverage? If yes, how long is it, and am I currently in the waiting period?
- If I am no longer able to work, is there an option to continue insurance coverage, such as through a COBRA policy? If yes, what

would my premiums be? How long would I be eligible for this coverage?

Keep in mind that regardless of how much your insurance covers, you'll be responsible for any costs not paid by your insurance. You can request an estimate of your out-of-pocket expenses from your transplant care team. Some insurance companies give you an estimate as well.

Patient advocates

Some hospitals and insurance companies employ what are called patient advocates. These individuals advocate on behalf of patients when issues arise or to make sure patients receive services they're entitled to. A patient advocate can be a useful resource if you hit a roadblock or need to dispute something with your health insurance company.

Ask your social worker or your financial coordinator about the availability of patient advocate services. You also can look for a patient advocate online at the Patient Advocate Foundation's website (see the Additional resources section at the end of this book).

MEDICATION COSTS

You'll need to work out the details of how you'll pay for the medications you must take immediately after surgery, including antirejection medications. Some of the medications will become lifelong medicines. Depending on your prescription coverage, this could be a substantial cost.

In the past, many antirejection medications were expensive and could add up to several thousand dollars a month. Now, many of the brand-name medications have generic alternatives. Generic drugs have the same active ingredients as brand-name drugs but cost less. The U.S. Food and Drug Administration rates generic and brand-name medications equally safe and effective. Generic medications typically have copays, but they're usually not very expensive.

If you must use brand-name medications, you may be able to take advantage of a copay card. A copay card is a coupon offered by the drug manufacturer to lower out-of-pocket costs on some brand-name medications. These are called copay assistance cards or copay savings programs. Ask your social worker or financial coordinator about copay cards.

Medicare covers transplant medications, but to receive benefits, you must join the plan's prescription coverage, called Medicare Part D. The amount of coverage also is dependent on whether you have Medicare Advantage or Original Medicare plus a Medigap plan.

A social worker can help you understand your medication coverage before your transplant, so you can be prepared to start medications immediately after surgery.

TRAVEL AND LODGING EXPENSES

If you don't live near a transplant center, you need to consider travel and lodging for yourself and your caregiver. A social worker can go over your travel and lodging options during your evaluation and may suggest steps to minimize these expenses or provide tips for getting reimbursed.

Before and during surgery

In the early stages of your transplant journey, you and your caregiver will likely travel to one or more transplant centers for evaluation, which may take up to a week and sometimes longer. If you choose to be evaluated at several different hospitals to increase your chances of receiving your transplant faster, you may take multiple trips and incur greater expenses. These costs can add up quickly.

If you live far from your chosen transplant center, you may decide to temporarily relocate nearby, depending on your medical condition, your position on the waiting list and the distance from your home to the center. Being near your transplant center can make it easier to get there and into the operating room more quickly.

During recovery

After you're discharged, you and your caregiver likely will need to remain near your hospital during your recovery. How long depends on the type of organ you received and how well you're recovering, but plan on at least a few weeks. For example, a typical recovery for liver

TRANSPLANT COSTS AT A GLANCE

If you have insurance, you typically pay out of your own pocket until you meet your plan's deductible, and then you pay a percentage of the costs or a copay for services including:

- Transplant evaluation and testing.
- Visits and consultations with surgeons, physicians, radiologists, anesthesiologists and other medical professionals.
- Laboratory tests.
- Recovery of the organ from the donor.
- Transplant surgery.
- Follow-up care and lab tests.
- Additional hospital stays if needed.
- Antirejection medications and other medicines.
- Rehabilitation, such as physical therapy.

Nonmedical costs, which may or may not be covered by insurance, may include:

- Lodging and travel expenses for you and your caregiver before, during and after transplant. This may include plane travel to get to your transplant hospital quickly when the donated organ becomes available.
- Child care during the time you and your caregiver are away.
- Car rental, ride-hailing services such as Uber and Lyft, or public transportation during your recovery.
- Any lost wages if your employer or your caregiver's employer cannot cover extended sick leave or family leave.

If you choose to be evaluated at several transplant centers, you'll have expenses at each location.

A VISIT WITH MAYO CLINIC TRANSPLANT CENTER
SOCIAL WORKER JENNA M. ROSENBERG, M.S.W., L.M.S.W.

Jenna M. Rosenberg, M.S.W., L.M.S.W., is a transplant social worker. Rosenberg regularly talks with people undergoing a transplant evaluation, and part of her job is to help them understand and prepare for the financial aspects of their journey.

"When people come in, we discuss the logistical aspects of transplant, such as finances and insurance. We assess if there are any financial barriers that we should address. For example, people may not realize that they may need to temporarily relocate to be closer to the clinic before their transplant, or they may not realize that they will have to stay near the hospital for several weeks during recovery."

Rosenberg says many people travel long distances to seek a transplant because transplant medicine isn't always available where they live. And for some people, travel and lodging is a concern because it's an upfront expense. Hospital bills will come later and may be broken down into a payment plan, but lodging is an immediate concern. "We work with people and their caregivers to help them plan ahead," says Rosenberg.

and kidney transplants takes 4 to 6 weeks, and a typical heart and lung transplant recovery, 8 to 12 weeks. Your transplant care team lets you know how much recovery time you may need based on your medical condition and the type of transplant you're having.

Coverage and reimbursements

Many private insurance plans offer coverage for travel, lodging and even food, but you may need to pay first and seek reimbursement later. Original Medicare doesn't pay for travel or lodging, but some Medicare Advantage plans may offer coverage.

Even when your plan covers these expenses, be prepared for caveats, such as reimbursement timelines and limits. For example, it

She also helps people explore insurance reimbursement options and understand insurance maximums or caps. "Let's say the lodging cap insurance will pay you is $100 per day, and you found a hotel that you want for $150," Rosenberg says. "So, $50 a day will come out of your own pocket. That's a financial expense that's still going to add up." She encourages people to be mindful of these kinds of details.

While waiting for a transplant, sometimes people relocate to be closer to their clinic. This can simplify logistics when the call comes through with an offer of an organ. For some, it may make sense to stay nearby for two or three months prior to transplant.

"We also make sure our patients can afford their medications after transplant," says Rosenberg. "We show people which medications are usually used after transplant, so that they can go to their insurance company and ask, 'What's my coverage for these medications?' Luckily, many transplant medications are now generic, and commercial insurance companies pay for them pretty well, so it's less of a concern than it was in the past."

may take 1 to 3 months to get reimbursed, depending on your insurance plan. In addition, most insurance companies have reimbursement maximums or caps. Some caps may have a lifetime maximum, and others, per-day limits.

Some transplant centers offer free or low-cost hospitality houses specifically for people receiving transplants. Be sure to ask your social worker about these options.

To offset expenses, you may be able to claim a portion of your medical-related travel, transportation and lodging costs as deductions on your personal tax return. An accountant or other tax professional can help you understand how to deduct these expenses properly. You also can search online for IRS Publication 502, Medical and Dental

Expenses, which explains how to claim them on your Schedule A tax form.

FOR CAREGIVERS: THE FINANCIAL IMPACT

Most transplant programs require a caregiver to be present 24 hours a day, seven days a week during the recovery period. Because of this, caregivers often need to ask for a leave of absence or a family leave from work. Depending on the circumstances, some programs also request a backup caregiver. This person generally doesn't need to take off work if the primary caregiver is present with the transplant recipient most of the time.

While most employers have policies allowing extended leave, some may not. If necessary, the social worker on your loved one's transplant care team often can write a letter to your employer explaining your situation, why your presence is required around the clock, and the length of time you'll need to take off work.

As part of a transplant evaluation, each patient receives a psychosocial assessment with a licensed transplant social worker. It's beneficial that you be present as well, to discuss any concerns and needs you may have. Share as much information as you can.

When meeting with your social worker:

- Prepare your questions in advance and write down the answers.
- Provide as much detail as possible when filling out the forms.
- Share your concerns or fears.
- Discuss what insurance covers and what it doesn't.
- Find out whether you'll have access to a patient advocate.
- Ask about the possibility of fundraising or getting help from advocacy organizations.
- If needed, ask for help in planning time off from work or arranging for child care during the transplant procedure and recovery periods.
- Ask about support groups.

4

When a child needs a transplant

A MOM'S BIGGEST GIFT
KENDON AND LISA'S STORY

More than a decade later, Lisa still remembers the fateful Friday night in 2012 that changed everything. A mother of three, Lisa was cooking dinner when her phone rang displaying the number of her son's pediatrician. "It was after hours, so I thought it was a little weird," Lisa recalls. But she couldn't have imagined what she was about to hear.

"I just wanted to let you know that we got Kendon's lab results back," the doctor told her. "His kidney numbers are not right, and they're a little concerning to me," the doctor continued. He then said that he had called ahead to a local hospital and Kendon "should probably go *now*."

Lisa had taken Kendon to the doctor's office two days earlier — not because he was sick but because of his grandmother's concern. Kendon's grandparents were visiting to attend his Boy Scouts Eagle Court of

Honor, and his grandmother observed that Kendon didn't look right. "I think it's because he's tired," Lisa told her mom. "He's a teenager."

Kendon indeed had a busy life. He had just started high school. His schedule changed so he had to get up early in the morning. He was taking honors classes and playing soccer. He did feel tired all the time but didn't think much of it. "I was pretty busy and adjusting to waking up early," Kendon recalls. "I just attributed all of my tiredness and my general fatigue to my lifestyle."

Lisa heeded her mom's concern and made an appointment for Kendon to see a doctor, who suspected mononucleosis, a viral infection that afflicts some teenagers and generally isn't overly concerning. But lab results showed that Kendon was dealing with something much more serious.

At the hospital, after a battery of tests, a nephrologist delivered the diagnosis. Kendon had oligomeganephronia, a rare congenital kidney malformation that affects how the kidneys function. And while the condition could be managed with medicine for a time, Kendon eventually would need a new kidney to replace the function of his two damaged kidneys.

"It wasn't a question of 'if,' it was a question of 'when,'" Lisa says. "I cried. Kendon cried. We all cried. It was one of those moments when you realize life's just never going to be the same again."

For the next few years, Kendon did well on kidney medicines. "For the rest of high school, I feel like I lived a pretty normal life," he says. "But it was always there, hanging over me." Kendon's mother agrees. "For me, it never really went away," she says. "It was always in the back of my mind."

Kendon graduated high school and went on a two-year mission with his church, purposefully staying near Los Angeles, a city with a robust hospital system that he would need to visit periodically.

Then, in 2018, things took a turn. About two months after Kendon came home from his mission, he landed in the emergency room. "It was July, and I was planning on starting college," he says. But his blood counts were extremely high. He'd lost weight, felt constantly nauseous and couldn't eat anything. "We could go to Mayo Clinic with my husband's insurance, so that's what we did," Lisa says. Kendon was hospitalized to get him stable and then began the transplant evaluation process.

"With the transplant testing, you need to be sick enough to need the transplant and yet be healthy enough to receive the kidney and withstand surgery," Lisa says. Kendon was in that sweet spot. He could go on the transplant waiting list, but how long he'd have to wait wasn't known. If the wait was too long, he'd have to go on dialysis, which Kendon didn't want to do. "A nephrologist told us that if you can go straight to transplant, that's best for the kidney, and best for your health," Kendon recalls. The family also learned that a kidney from a living donor generally worked better and performed longer than a kidney from a deceased donor.

Lisa decided to be her son's living donor. "I think I always knew that it would be me," she says. Kendon's father and older sister didn't qualify for medical reasons, and his younger sister was only 16 so she couldn't donate. When the tests showed that Lisa was a match, she was relieved. "There was just something in the back of my mind that I just knew I was the one who was supposed to do it."

Mom and son were scheduled for surgery in September 2018. When their time came, Lisa went in first. Kendon followed, and within a few hours, he had his mother's kidney. "It could've still been warm when they put it in," Lisa says with a chuckle. "Afterward, his surgeon told us that as soon as they hooked up that kidney, it immediately started making urine. And his surgeon said it was the best thing he's ever seen."

Having a working kidney changed things instantly. "I woke up and I immediately felt like the weight had been lifted off me," Kendon recalls. He stopped feeling slow and sluggish. "I always felt like my blood was super thick — that's the best way I can describe it, just very sluggish and heavy. And I remember waking up in the hospital and not feeling that anymore."

As mom and son were recovering, Kendon's father took over managing Kendon's medicines, which was complex. "You had to take this medication every four hours, but that medication every six hours, and then this one once a day, and then these two twice a day," Kendon says. "And they were changing the doses every day that we would go in."

One night, after being concerned that he messed up the doses, and counting the remaining pills in various bottles, Kendon's father, an accountant, turned to spreadsheets to institute a system. "My medications became my father's domain," Kendon quips. "I was very lucky that my family were such great caregivers. I was four days postsurgery. I couldn't even sit up on my own. So I really relied very heavily on other people to help me."

The transplant worked, and in January 2019, Kendon started college. By then, he had his medicine regimen down and was adjusting to his new normal. "With transplant, you have to grow up pretty fast," Lisa says. "You can't have that normal teenage feeling of I'm invincible, I can do what I want, and nothing is going to hurt me. A transplant experience pushes you to the point where you really do have to face your own mortality."

Kendon became diligent about reading labels on every food product he bought and avoiding fruits such as pomegranate and grapefruit, which can affect how antirejection medicines work. "Some things I've learned the hard way," Kendon says. "Once, I ended up eating bean sprouts, which I can't eat. They were in a hot soup. It's been boiled. I was sure it was fine. And then I ended up having a six-month-long infection because of it."

Lisa learned some things the hard way too. Once she put a grapefruit-scented hand soap in the bathroom, and suddenly Kendon got concerning lab results. The family got a call asking whether Kendon was eating foods he should avoid. "Even grapefruit-scented soap affected his labs and his medication," Lisa says. "So from that point, we checked hand soap, laundry soap, anything."

The transplant experience spurred Kendon to a medical career as a doctor. He's thinking about becoming a urologist. He also hopes to improve access to medicines, so people like him don't have to spend hours on the phone with their medical insurance to get their medicines covered and delivered on time.

Recently, Kendon got married, which meant his wife needed to learn the nuances of living with a transplant, such as adhering to the diet, reading the labels and avoiding people who appear sick, to name a few. As Lisa watched her son beam with joy at the wedding ceremony, she was thrilled that she played a role in that. "There's part of me that was able to make him that happy," she says. A few years down the road, Kendon and his wife plan to start a family, so Lisa looks forward to being a grandmother one day too.

Today, Lisa serves on the executive board of the National Kidney Foundation of Arizona, working to spread awareness of the benefits of kidney transplants and alleviate people's fears of the process. "I wish someone would've done that for me," Lisa says. "Someone who would've said: 'Hey, listen, it's going to be so much better. Don't dread it so much. Don't be so scared of it. It's really not the end of somebody's life. It's actually your chance at a new beginning.'"

Learning that your child needs an organ transplant can trigger many intense emotions: heartbreak over such a serious diagnosis, fear of something going wrong during the complex surgery, uncertainty about your child's future.

These feelings are understandable as you and your child embark on what can best be described as a challenging journey. Yet, it's essential to keep your eye on the transplant goal: the opportunity for your child to not only survive but thrive. And the good news is, thanks to how organs are matched to recipients and improved transplant-related care, more children are living well with organ transplants.

This chapter will help you understand the early stages of the transplant process, with the hope of easing many of your concerns. A key element to remember is that while a transplant can cure your child's original illness, with a transplant comes the need for lifelong management. Transplant recipients must take medicine daily and continue to get routine checkups with their transplant team and primary care team. These new responsibilities are necessary to make sure the transplant doesn't fail (see Chapter 16).

If your child's healthcare team recommends a transplant, it's because the benefits of the surgery outweigh the risks involved in living with a transplanted organ.

EVALUATION

One of the first steps in the transplant journey is a thorough medical evaluation. This is done to make sure your child is a good candidate for an organ transplant. Factors such as the severity of the disease, your child's overall health, including other medical conditions, and whether the benefits outweigh the risks are carefully considered by a team of pediatric transplant specialists.

As part of the evaluation, the transplant team looks at the following factors:

- **Blood tests.** These tests help determine your child's blood type (see page 34) and provide insight into an organ's function, your child's nutritional status and whether your child has any active infections that could compromise a transplant. Blood tests also provide information about the levels and strength of specific antibodies in the blood. These antibodies may attack a transplanted organ and increase the risk of rejection. Certain antibodies can make it harder to find a donor match, which may increase the wait time for a donor organ.
- **Biopsy results.** Sometimes, a biopsy of the organ needing a transplant may be necessary for more in-depth evaluation.
- **Imaging.** X-rays, ultrasounds, MRIs and CT scans help visualize organ structure and blood flow.
- **Size.** The transplant team will note your child's body size to ensure the donor organ is the appropriate size for your child.
- **Vaccinations.** Ideally, your child should be up to date on childhood vaccinations before the transplant to prevent infections or illnesses that could compromise your child's health. Your transplant team may recommend specific vaccines prior to transplantation.
- **Support.** Educational resources and counseling are important to help your family prepare for transplantation's physical, emotional and social impacts.
- **Donor options.** After the evaluation, the transplant team will meet to discuss whether transplantation is the right approach for your child. If it is, the team will discuss how quickly your child needs a transplant and what donor options are available, including being placed on the transplant waiting list.

Things to consider

After your child is approved for a transplant, you'll have a lot to think about. A transplant is a big commitment, one that requires many appointments and tests, both before and after the procedure. The success of the transplant will rely on your child going to all scheduled appointments and having all the recommended tests.

Making sure your child receives antirejection medicines as prescribed is critical. You'll need to understand when and how to administer them. Your active participation and commitment to your child's care plan before and after a transplant are vital for a successful transplant.

Your child may be dealing with strong emotions about the transplant, especially if your child is older and can grasp what's happening. It can be daunting to think about undergoing transplant surgery and having to rely on a donor organ for many years, along with the possibility of going through surgery again later if the organ needs to be replaced.

It's also challenging to manage a lifelong medical condition. As older children take their first steps toward independence and take more responsibility for their health, they may be less careful about following treatment plans, such as taking their daily medicines. As the immune system grows stronger, it's more capable of triggering rejection, making antirejection medications even more important.

Rejection is what happens when the body's immune system reacts against the transplanted organ. This can lead to new organ failure. To prevent rejection, transplant recipients need to take medicine every day to suppress the body's immune system. Rejection may still happen, despite the use of medicine to prevent it. But if identified right away, a rejection episode usually can be treated successfully with additional medicines.

Antirejection medicines, also called immunosuppressants, aren't without side effects. These medicines can increase the risk of cancer, infection or damage to other organs. On the other hand, a young child is still developing. Not getting an organ transplant can seriously affect a child's health, leading to issues with growth, brain development and possible injury to other organs.

KIDNEY TRANSPLANT

A transplant can be a lifesaving procedure for children with end-stage kidney disease or kidney failure. Kidney failure means the kidneys can no longer filter waste and excess fluids from the blood.

If not treated, kidney disease can lead to many complications in children, including severe anemia, high blood pressure, issues with bone health, shorter height, delayed puberty and cognitive issues.

What a child understands about a transplant can depend on the experience up to this point. Children who've been otherwise healthy may not be accustomed to seemingly endless appointments and tests. For these children, the transplant process is likely to require a significant adjustment period. Other children may have had to navigate chronic diseases and frequent medical appointments for most of their lives. For them, the demands of the transplant process may feel relatively familiar.

Children old enough to understand what is happening may have questions about the transplant. Here are some common questions and suggestions for how you might respond.

Where does my new organ come from?

Your response to this question depends on the type of organ transplant. Hearts and lungs come from a deceased donor, while kidneys, livers and intestines can come from a deceased donor or a living donor. Here are a couple of options for how to respond, depending on the circumstance.

Your heart may come from someone who died suddenly, and that person's family has agreed to give it to a child like you who needs it.

Your liver might come from someone who's alive and who wants to give a part of their liver to help someone who needs one, like you. A liver grows back if part of it is taken out. That means that someone can give you a portion of liver. You'll feel better, and the other person will be OK too. Giving a portion of liver won't make the person sick.

Does the transplant hurt?

During the operation, you get a special medicine called anesthesia. It makes you sleep, so you do not feel anything during the operation. When the operation is over, you wake up. You may feel sore and uncomfortable after the operation. But you get medicine to help you feel better.

Could I die?
With any surgery, there's a tiny chance of dying. But this surgery gives you the best chance for a longer, better life.

Will I be the same person after the operation?
Yes. After you leave the hospital, you will still be you. But you'll feel stronger and healthier. When you start to feel better you can return to school, spend time with friends and have fun.

Will I have to do anything different after the transplant?
You'll need to take medicine every day for the rest of your life after the transplant. This is very important. When you get a new organ, your body doesn't know whether the organ is something good or something bad. If your body thinks the organ is something bad, your body tries to attack the organ. The medicine keeps your body from fighting your new organ. That keeps you healthy. You'll also need to see your doctor every so often and have tests to make sure everything is good.

Is it OK to be afraid?
Yes, it's OK to be afraid. Do you want to talk about what you are afraid of? I can try to help you understand what is making you feel scared, and so can your doctors, nurses and other people at the hospital. You can ask them questions too. Or you can ask me, and I can ask the questions for you.

When children are afraid, they need information, love and support. Be honest with your child, but also try to be reassuring.

Why is a kidney transplant needed?

There are many possible causes of chronic kidney disease and kidney failure in children that require a kidney transplant. These include:

- **Congenital conditions.** A child may be born without fully developed kidneys or with an obstruction that leads urine to back up, resulting in kidney damage.
- **Genetic conditions.** A child can inherit a condition that damages the kidneys. For example, polycystic kidney disease is an inherited condition that causes cyst growth in the kidneys.
- **Infections.** Bacteria can trigger serious conditions that prevent the kidneys from working correctly. For example, an infection caused by certain strains of *E. coli* can cause a condition called hemolytic uremic syndrome, which can lead to kidney failure.
- **Nephrotic syndrome.** Conditions such as focal glomerulosclerosis, which causes the body to pass too much protein in urine, can damage the tiny filters in the kidneys.
- **Systemic diseases.** Autoimmune diseases such as lupus can attack the kidneys.
- **Trauma.** Injuries, dehydration, burns and other trauma can cause low blood pressure and decreased blood flow to the kidneys, resulting in kidney failure.
- **Urine reflux or blockages.** Urine that backs up to the kidneys can lead to kidney infections and damage.

Of these causes, congenital conditions, genetic conditions and nephrotic syndrome are some of the most common.

Dialysis versus transplant

To treat kidney failure, there are two options: dialysis and kidney transplant. Dialysis is a treatment that uses a machine to perform the functions of the kidneys, removing waste from the bloodstream, keeping fluid and mineral levels in check, and helping to stabilize blood pressure. However, it's usually considered a temporary solution.

Kidney transplantation is usually the preferred treatment for children. Children who undergo transplants have better survival rates and quality of life than children who stay on dialysis. About half of children who receive a kidney transplant will reach a typical height.

Receiving a kidney

Children are more likely than adults to undergo what's called a preemptive kidney transplant. This means that a transplant, not dialysis, is their first line of treatment. Generally, this means a child will still be in relatively good health at the time of the transplant. Some research has found improved survival in children who receive a preemptive kidney transplant.

There's also the benefit of avoiding health issues and dietary restrictions associated with dialysis. Getting a kidney transplant earlier also may prevent some of the complications caused by kidney disease, such as shorter height and delayed puberty.

With a preemptive kidney transplant, a child typically receives a kidney from a living donor, often from a family member or friend. Paired donation can help make living donation possible if a child has a potential living donor who's not a match for them. A paired kidney donation, also known as a kidney exchange, is a transplant option that allows two or more pairs of living donors to exchange kidneys to create compatible matches. If a living donor isn't available, a child can be placed on the waitlist for a deceased donor and may be able to receive a kidney before needing dialysis.

Not everyone is a candidate for a preemptive transplant. Overall health, certain conditions and ongoing infections can prevent a person from moving straight to transplant. Your child's transplant team is the best source of information on whether a preemptive transplant is an option.

If your child isn't a candidate for a preemptive transplant, the next step usually will be to begin dialysis treatment and plan for transplant to happen at a later time — either from a living donor or from a deceased donor. How long your child has to wait depends on the availability of a kidney and finding the right match. However, those under age 18 are given priority on kidney transplant waitlists.

HEART TRANSPLANT

Heart transplantation is performed for children who have heart failure. Heart failure means the heart muscle doesn't pump blood as well as it should. When this happens, blood often backs up, and fluid can build up in the lungs, causing shortness of breath.

In children, heart failure most often is caused by either a structural heart issue they were born with or by cardiomyopathy, which causes the heart to have a harder time pumping blood to the rest of the body. Heart failure can lead to complications such as blood clots, dangerous irregular heartbeats called arrhythmias and sudden cardiac death.

A transplant often is a last resort for children after other treatment options have failed. It also may be an option for those experiencing severe medication side effects, such as an inability to be active or growth issues. A transplant procedure replaces a failing heart with a heart from a deceased child donor. The transplant gives the recipient an opportunity for extended life and improved health. This heart typically will grow to adult size as the child grows.

Why is a heart transplant needed?

Cardiomyopathies are a leading cause of heart failure and transplant in children. They include:

- **Dilated cardiomyopathy.** This is the most common form of cardiomyopathy linked to heart failure. It is characterized by an enlarged and weakened heart muscle.
- **Hypertrophic cardiomyopathy.** With this condition, the heart muscle thickens, obstructing blood flow.
- **Restrictive cardiomyopathy.** With this condition, the heart muscle becomes rigid, impairing the heart's ability to fill with blood. This condition is rare.

Severe congenital heart conditions may require transplantation if other surgical treatments aren't possible. These include:

- **Hypoplastic left heart syndrome.** In this condition, the left side of the heart isn't developed enough to pump enough blood to the body successfully.
- **Transposition of the great arteries.** In this condition, the main arteries leaving the heart are reversed.

MECHANICAL CIRCULATORY SUPPORT

While your child waits for a donor heart to become available, mechanical circulatory support can help maintain the remaining organ function and reduce the heart's oxygen requirements. Options include:

- **Ventricular assist device (VAD).** A VAD is a mechanical pump implanted in your child's chest that helps pump blood from the lower chambers of the heart to the rest of the body. Currently, VAD options are limited in smaller children.
- **Extracorporeal membrane oxygenation (ECMO).** ECMO is used for children who are at high risk of cardiac arrest or those who have had cardiac arrest. The device bypasses the heart and lungs to provide full heart and lung support for days or weeks. ECMO may serve as a bridge to using a VAD.

Mechanical circulatory support also may be used as a long-term treatment for an older person who isn't a transplant candidate.

Other conditions that may result in the need for transplantation include heart tumors, myocarditis and certain arrhythmias that don't respond to treatment.

Receiving a heart

Hearts from deceased children and adolescents whose families have agreed to donation are matched first to those children in the local area. That's followed by a search for a match in the region and then at the national level.

If your child is under the age of 1 and in need of a heart transplant, an ABO-incompatible transplant may be an option. This is a transplant in which a donor heart can have any blood type because an infant's immune system is very immature and less likely to reject it.

LIVER TRANSPLANT

A liver transplant may be considered if your child's liver has failed or if your child has a disease that can be treated with a transplant. Many forms of liver disease may be treated with a transplant, including certain forms of liver cancer.

Liver failure can lead to complications such as jaundice, issues with brain function, bleeding, abdominal swelling and kidney damage.

LESS COMMON TRANSPLANTS IN CHILDREN

Though not as common as other types of transplants, it's possible to transplant intestines or lungs to help children survive or to treat a chronic condition.

Intestinal transplant

Intestinal transplants can come from deceased or living donors, though deceased-donor organs are more common. Intestinal transplantation is a critical procedure for children with severe intestinal failure. Intestinal failure leads to the inability of the intestines to absorb necessary nutrients and fluids. It can be caused by:

- **Short bowel syndrome.** This condition is caused by surgery on large portions of the bowels or because of congenital conditions such as necrotizing enterocolitis and volvulus. It is the most common reason for intestinal transplant.
- **Intestinal motility conditions.** These include conditions that affect how food moves through the bowels, such as chronic intestinal pseudo-obstruction.
- **Congenital enterocyte conditions.** Conditions such as microvillus inclusion disease or tufting enteropathy cause severe, chronic diarrhea.
- **Parenteral therapy complications.** Parenteral therapy bypasses the digestive system to provide nutrition to children through

Why is a liver transplant needed?

Liver transplantation is used to treat several conditions:

- **Biliary atresia.** This is the most common reason for liver transplant in young people. It's a condition in which a newborn's bile ducts are blocked or absent.
- **Metabolic liver diseases.** Conditions such as Wilson's disease, alpha-1-antitrypsin deficiency and urea cycle disorders can damage the liver.

an IV. Complications may include liver disease, catheter infections and blood clots.

Lung transplant

Lung transplants for children usually rely on organs from deceased donors. Lung transplantation may be the best choice for children with end-stage lung disease who have exhausted all other treatment options. Common causes of end-stage lung disease in children include:

- **Cystic fibrosis.** An inherited disease characterized by chronic lung infections and progressive lung damage, it's the most common reason for lung transplantation in children.
- **Pulmonary hypertension.** This condition is a result of high blood pressure in the arteries of the lungs.
- **Interstitial lung disease.** Chronic lung inflammation brought on by interstitial lung disease can cause the lungs to become scarred and stiff.
- **Bronchiolitis obliterans.** This condition can produce severe infection or lung injury that can damage and scar the smallest airways in the lungs.

- **Acute liver failure.** Infections, toxins, medicines or autoimmune diseases can cause the liver to stop working suddenly without any history of prior liver issues.
- **Cystic fibrosis.** This inherited disease causes the body to produce thick mucus, which clogs bile ducts and leads to inflammation that damages the liver. This disease also commonly affects the lungs.
- **Chronic liver disease.** Hepatitis and certain genetic conditions can lead to liver damage called cirrhosis.

Though rare in children, cancerous tumors such as hepatoblastoma also may require a liver transplant.

Determining urgency

Unlike other diseases, such as kidney failure in which kidney dialysis can help compensate for the damaged organ, liver failure can only be treated with a transplant. A scoring system is used to determine priority on the transplant waiting list. Healthcare professionals use the Model for End-Stage Liver Disease (MELD) score for transplant candidates age 12 and older and the Pediatric End-Stage Liver Disease (PELD) score for those younger than 12.

Your child's healthcare team will use a specific formula to determine a score. The score estimates the risk of death within 90 days without a transplant. A high score indicates an urgent need for a transplant.

As deceased-donor organs become available, they're classified by blood type and given to recipients according to scores. Candidates with higher scores generally are offered donated livers first. Time spent on the liver transplant waiting list is used to aid in decisions among candidates with the same scores and blood types.

Some candidates may have medical conditions, such as liver cancer, that may not accurately reflect their transplant need. In these cases, they may get a separate score or be exempted and placed higher on the transplant waiting list.

Receiving a liver

Donor livers can come from deceased or living donors. A deceased donor's organ must match your child's size and blood type, though sometimes a deceased donor liver can be reduced in size. The wait for a donor liver can vary greatly, and depends on the MELD or PELD score, as well as blood type. Some people wait days, while others wait months or may never receive a deceased donor's liver.

A living donor is usually a relative, such as a parent or other relative, or a close family friend. Living-donor transplants typically involve removing a portion of the donor's liver, which then regenerates over time. Living-donor liver transplants can reduce the wait time, which can reduce the risk of issues that may result from prolonged time on the waiting list.

In some cases, a full liver from a deceased donor may be split into two parts to implant in a child and an adult awaiting transplant. Research suggests this approach could help reduce the number of children who die waiting for a liver.

WHAT LIES AHEAD

If your child has to wait for a donor organ, your emotions will likely be headed into new territory. You may experience concern about your child's health deteriorating if the wait is long, dismay about any setbacks, and an intense hope that the next call you get brings news that a donor has been found.

The wait is often unpredictable, lasting days, weeks, months or even years, depending on the type of transplant your child needs. Sometimes, a donor organ isn't found. All of this uncertainty about what lies ahead can leave you emotionally drained.

Chapter 8 covers what to expect when you have a child on the transplant waitlist. Understanding this part of the journey can help you feel more prepared and empowered while waiting for that life-changing gift.

5

Finding a donor

REACHING OUT FOR HELP
STEVEN'S STORY

Ask Steven whether he considers himself a lucky guy, and he'll give you an immediate "Yes!" While some people may think that life dealt them a blow in the form of failing kidneys, Steven thinks he was blessed on many counts. "I'm very fortunate," he says, always one to look on the positive side of things. "And I'm very grateful too."

Steven was 55 when an imaging test he was doing for a routine checkup revealed he had polycystic kidney disease, a genetic disorder that causes fluid-filled cysts to form in the kidneys. Steven was neither overly surprised nor very scared. His mother also had polycystic kidney disease, and she lived to age 98. The diagnosis did, however, explain certain health issues he was having, such as high blood pressure and swollen ankles caused by his body retaining extra fluid. Occasionally, a cyst would burst, causing a lot of pain and making him urinate blood.

Still, for the next 13 years, Steven's kidneys functioned well enough that he could go on with his life. "I was under nephrology care, where they were doing quarterly blood tests to see how the disease was progressing," he says. Then, in July 2020, Steven's kidney function declined to the point his nephrologist said he'd need a transplant. By November, Steven was on the waiting list, but his transplant coordinator suggested looking for a living donor for a better outcome and shorter wait time. The coordinator advised casting a very wide net to see who may respond.

Steven wasn't comfortable asking friends and family to donate a kidney. So instead, he started telling people about his situation. "I don't know if I was just timid or embarrassed. So what I did do is make phone calls to some people I'm very close with to inform them about what was going on in my life." To his surprise, all of them said they wanted to test to find out whether they could be donors. "I had eight people sign up to be tested," Steven says.

Not everyone passed the donor test, but Steven's childhood friend Mark did. He was healthy enough to donate a kidney. There was only one issue. Steven and Mark had different blood types. That meant that Steven's immune system would immediately reject Mark's kidney.

When that happens, transplant teams organize what are called paired donations, in which they find another nonmatching donor-recipient pair that can be cross-matched. In such paired donations, each recipient gets a compatible organ. The search took some time, but by August 2021, Steven was scheduled for his surgery.

Everything fell into place. A couple Steven and his wife knew offered them their winter house so they could be close to the hospital. "I was very lucky," Steven says.

The surgery went well. "Mark was in the hospital for a day, and I was in the hospital for two," Steven recalls. The donated kidney worked right away. "I remember my wife came up to see me and said, 'Oh my God, your ankles aren't swollen!'" Soon both friends were home, recovering together, and taking long walks in the early mornings. Managing medicines was a challenge, but Steven's wife, Linda, took charge. "Linda is a perfectionist, which is actually a good thing when it comes to medications," Steven says.

Four months after his transplant, Steven encountered an unexpected hurdle. "I was back at Mayo for 16 days because I had a rejection event," he says. He knew it as soon as he saw his routine lab results. "By then, I've read enough labs to know that there was a major problem. They put me straight back into the hospital," he says. After his transplant team adjusted his medicines, he was back home again. "From that point on, I live what I call my new normal, which is a really great life. I play golf. I exercise. I travel. I get on an airplane. I've been to Europe. We now have a grandchild. I have a lot of things to be grateful for."

Support groups helped Steven and Linda prepare and cope, so once he was on the mend, he volunteered to help others undergoing a transplant journey. "I'm a mentor. I give back. I talk to pretransplant patients who need some guidance," he says. His topmost advice to those beginning their transplant journey is staying healthy, fit and positive. "You've got to surround yourself with positive people and eliminate negativity from your life," he says. "I went into it with a positive attitude. I trusted the doctors. I trusted the science. And it all worked out."

Transplantation is possible because of people who choose to donate their organs. And it's important to remember that organ donors are not a select group. People of all ages and medical backgrounds can become donors.

TYPES OF DONORS

There are basically two types of organ donors. Those who choose to donate their organs when they die, and those who do so while they're still living. In either case, a donated organ can be lifesaving for the recipient.

Deceased donors

Most organs that are donated for transplantation come from deceased donors who have sustained a severe injury — often after a stroke, heart attack or a serious accident — that led to brain death. If a person has indicated a willingness to be an organ donor, such as on a driver's license, or if the family thinks that donation is what their loved one would have wanted, the process of donation begins. Eventually, an operation is performed to remove and preserve the person's organs so they can be transplanted into people in need of a new organ.

In some situations, such as after a severe injury, a person may be on life support. If there is no hope of recovery, families must decide whether to withdraw life support from a loved one. When making this decision, families also may decide to pursue organ donation. Life support is removed near or in the operating room. After the heart stops beating and the person experiences cardiac death, surgery is performed to remove and preserve the organs. This is called donation after circulatory death (DCD).

Living donors

Some organ donations come from living donors. Because it's possible to lead a healthy life with just one kidney, a person who is living can donate a kidney. After kidney donation, the remaining kidney increases in size and takes care of filtering waste all on its own. Some kidney donors say that their quality of life has improved because they saved somebody else's life.

Similarly, you can donate a part of your liver. The human liver can quickly regenerate back to its original size both in the donor and in the recipient.

Living donors enabled more than 7,000 transplants in 2024 in the United States. This lifesaving procedure is more important than ever because of the rising need for organs and the shortage of organs from deceased donors.

You can learn more about being a living donor in the next chapter.

TRANSPLANT ORGANIZATIONS

Organ donation and transplantation is a complex process that requires the expertise and collaboration of many people. These are some organizations that play key roles in organ donation.

Organ procurement and transplantation network

The Organ Procurement and Transplantation Network (OPTN) is a partnership between public and private institutions that oversees the national organ transplant system. The network links all medical professionals involved in transplant in the U.S. It has a board of directors and committees that develop and oversee rules and policies governing the transplant system.

When you envision an organ transplant, you might picture a medical professional running, cooler in hand, to transport an organ to a recipient as fast as possible. Though this scenario still exists, a new image has come into view. Instead of using ice, organs to be transplanted are kept "alive" and functioning outside of the body by machine perfusion technology.

With this new technology, an organ travels in a specialized chamber, like a box, that pumps warm, oxygenated blood into the organ. The blood delivers nutrients and other substances the organ needs to remain fully functioning outside of the body. Kidneys have been transported using a similar device for many years. The technology has now advanced to support the transport of hearts and livers.

Machine perfusion can extend the time between retrieval and transport of an organ by several hours. It also widens the donor pool, and shortens recipients' waiting time, by allowing transplant teams to use organs that might not have sustained cold storage, as well as organs that previously might not have been usable.

For example, a heart that stops beating after circulatory death cannot be donated using standard cold storage methods. But machine perfusion can revive the heart from nonbeating to beating status, allowing for a successful donation after circulatory death (DCD). In addition, the perfusion system measures and analyzes the heart's function in real time, allowing the transplant team to confirm whether it's indeed acceptable for transplant.

Lungs also can be kept functioning outside the body through what's called ex vivo lung perfusion (EVLP). Such a system can evaluate the health and status of donated lungs, as well as preserve them during unforeseen delays. In the future, specialists hope to improve the quality of donated lungs by providing medicines or cell therapies during EVLP.

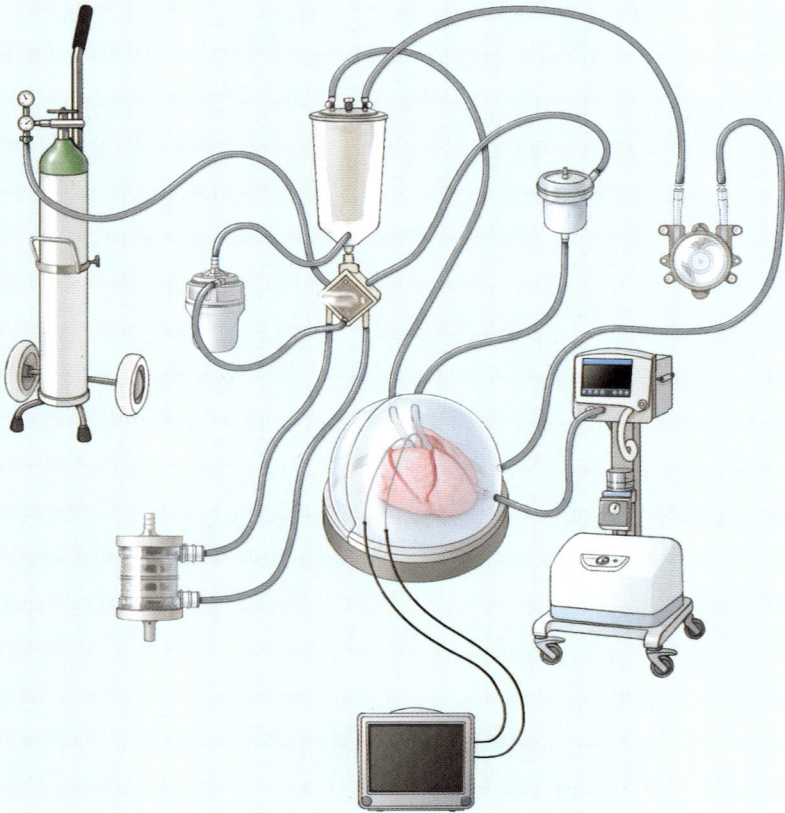

With ex vivo lung perfusion (EVLP), removed donor lungs are placed in a specialized chamber. Inside, a protein-rich solution and gases are circulated through the lungs to reduce swelling and remove excess fluid. This technology allows for preservation and even restoration of function of less healthy lungs. It also can help transplant care teams determine whether a donor lung will work properly in a recipient.

United network for organ sharing

United Network for Organ Sharing (UNOS) is a nonprofit scientific and educational organization that is contracted to operate OPTN. It uses a computer system to match recipients and donors. The system takes into account the recipient's order on the waitlist as well as details that determine whether the organ is a match for the recipient.

UNOS follows policies developed by the OPTN. Depending on which organ is needed, order on the waitlist may differ, though many of the same principles apply. The system continuously looks for matches to maximize the chances of successful transplantation.

Organ procurement organizations

Organ procurement organizations (OPOs) are nonprofit organizations responsible for managing organ donors and coordinating organ recoveries so that organs get to awaiting transplant candidates. There are more than 50 OPOs in the United States.

In many cases, transplant surgeons travel to the medical center where the donor is located to procure organs for their patients. However, local surgeons from the OPO or a nearby transplant center also may perform the organ recovery operation.

You won't work directly with UNOS or an OPO. Your transplant care team will work with these organizations on your behalf to find you the best match in the shortest possible time.

More information on these and other transplant organizations is listed in the Additional resources section at the end of the book.

GETTING LISTED

Once you've completed a transplant evaluation and are eligible for an organ transplant, you can choose to be placed on the national transplant waiting list. Your transplant center will register you. It's possible to be listed at more than one transplant center, which may be helpful in getting a transplant faster, depending on your medical condition and the resources you have available to travel.

Once you're listed, your data will be entered into the UNOS computerized matching system. The matching process depends on your position on the waitlist as well as the organ you are waiting for.

For example, the liver waiting list is determined according to urgency — the sickest people are at the top of the list. Prioritization on the liver list is calculated by the MELD score (see pages 44-45). People who need a kidney are prioritized using a combination of factors, including waiting time as well as other factors such as the EPTS score, and whether the recipient has antibodies against human leukocyte antigen, also known as HLA (see pages 34-35), which can make the kidneys hard to match. In addition, donor organ distribution also considers the transplant hospital's location relative to the donor's hospital.

When a match becomes available for you, an offer is made to your transplant center. Your surgeon and the transplant team will review the offer to make sure it's the right organ for you. If it is, they'll call you to see whether you accept the offer.

MAXIMIZING YOUR CHANCES

The wait for a donated organ can be long, but there are a few things you can do to shorten your wait time.

Stay close to your transplant hospital

When organs become available, they must be transplanted within a matter of hours. When the UNOS system locates a match, you'll need to get to the transplant hospital quickly. Depending on your position on the waitlist and your medical condition, your transplant center may ask you to temporarily live closer to the hospital so you can arrive for a transplant in a timely manner.

Consider a living donor for kidney and liver transplants

Waiting for a deceased-donor organ that's compatible can take a long time — sometimes months and even years. If you need a kidney or liver transplant, receiving a kidney or a portion of a liver from a living donor is another option. If you have a relative or a friend who is willing to donate, that could significantly shorten your waiting time. It also could reduce the chances of medical problems occurring while you're waiting for transplantation. A living donor also may allow you to get a high-quality donor organ. (You can read more about being a living donor in the next chapter.)

There's a chance that you may not be compatible with your living donor. In this case, your transplant care team will check into what's called paired donation. A paired exchange is a process that allows incompatible donor-recipient pairs to exchange donors to create compatible matches, in which the donor of each pair is compatible with the recipient of the other pair. If both donors and recipients are willing, the transplant care team will proceed with such a paired-organ donation. In some cases, paired donations may include several pairs.

List at multiple hospitals

To boost your chances of getting a transplant, consider listing at more than one hospital. OPTN policies allow you to be listed at multiple locations.

If you decide to be listed in several hospitals, you need to go through the evaluation process at each location. Different hospitals may use different listing criteria. Check with your insurance provider to see whether visits and tests at multiple medical centers are covered. (See Chapter 3 for more on the financial aspects of transplantation.) Also, keep in mind the distance between you and the hospitals.

SOLVING THE ORGAN SHORTAGE PROBLEM

There are more than 100,000 people on the transplant waiting list. Every eight minutes another name is added. Some people wait for months and years for a transplant, and some die before they can receive a new organ. Living donation can be a solution for people who are waiting for a liver or a kidney. But it's not an option for people waiting for other organs, and not everyone has a suitable donor. Because of the shortage of available organs, scientists are exploring new ways to solve the problem.

Bioartificial livers

Several types of bioartificial livers — devices that perform liver functions for people with liver failure — have been developed in recent years. Mayo Clinic is refining its own version of a bioartificial liver, known as the Spheroid Reservoir Bioartificial Liver (SRBAL). Similar to kidney dialysis, it functions outside a person's body, using pig or human

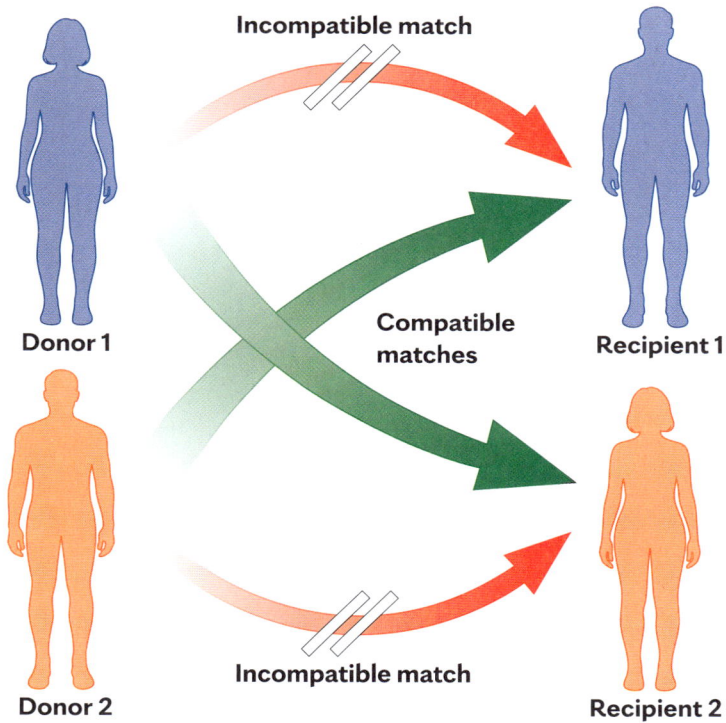

Incompatible match

Compatible matches

Incompatible match

Donor 1 — Recipient 1

Donor 2 — Recipient 2

In a paired kidney donation, the donor of one pair of people is compatible with the recipient of another pair of people. If all parties are willing to undergo the exchange, both recipients benefit from a new organ.

liver cells to filter blood. The goal is that the device can avoid the need for a liver transplant by supporting an injured liver as it heals and regenerates itself. The device also may help people with end-stage liver disease manage their condition while they await a transplant.

Tissue engineering

One of the questions transplant researchers are asking is, "Could we bioengineer organs to reduce or eliminate the waitlist?" To answer that question, Mayo Clinic has formed a collaboration with Carnegie

People in need of a transplant from medically underserved communities — those who lack medical insurance or who live in rural areas, for example — oftentimes face challenges to receiving a needed organ transplant. They may be diagnosed at a later stage and tend to arrive for transplant evaluation sicker than people who seek evaluation earlier. They may need to travel farther for their appointments and may not always have the means to get there. And some may not have a caregiver to accompany them throughout the transplant process.

People with fewer resources also may face difficulties navigating the complex evaluation process or understanding why they need a transplant. To help them through their transplant journey, Mayo Clinic in Arizona recently launched a new initiative called Boldly Promoting Health Equity Through Novel Transplant Patient Navigator Services.

The initiative was prompted by the case of a Navajo man who was referred for a liver transplant even though he didn't know that he had liver cancer. The initiative aims to solve some of the challenges facing minority populations by offering extra help. With this program, a member of the Native American community serves as a guide and an interpreter throughout the evaluation process. A similar program is being developed at Mayo Clinic in Minnesota. Other transplant programs also offer programs geared to meet the needs of specific underserved populations.

Because certain health conditions that can result in the need for a transplant, such as kidney or heart disease, are more common in African American, Hispanic and Native American communities, UNOS also is working to improve the transplant allocation system to reduce inequities.

Mellon University, pairing medical expertise with engineering know-how to create experimental organs.

"Bioengineering new organs is promising, but complex. We're looking at a research timeline of 10 to 15 years to potentially bring this new option to patients," says C. Burcin Taner, M.D., who leads the Transforming Transplant Initiative at Mayo Clinic in collaboration with Mayo Clinic's Center for Regenerative Biotherapeutics.

The bioengineering research brings together 3D bioprinting, tissue engineering, biomaterials and cellular materials to grow humanlike organs. The research focuses on a range of areas, from better ways of monitoring the health of transplanted organs to engineering complex organs such as hearts, lungs, livers and kidneys. Many other healthcare professionals and scientists are working on tissue engineering to address the organ shortage worldwide, and promising discoveries are being made.

Xenotransplantation
Human-to-human transplantation is complex, but animal-to-human transplantation, also called xenotransplantation, is even more challenging. For starters, animal organs and human organs must match in size. The most suitable animals size-wise are pigs. But pigs are genetically different from humans. They also have very different antigens on their cells, making it difficult to avoid organ rejection.

However, today's genetic technologies offer hope. Thanks to genetic engineering, scientists can now "knock out" the most problematic antigens on pig cells. While this progress is promising, the next step is to perform a human trial to gather important information and learn more about the safety and function of pig organs. Clinical trials for transplanting pig kidneys in humans are being designed now.

Researchers and scientists hope that innovations such as tissue engineering and xenotransplantation eventually can become a viable option so that more people can receive transplanted organs.

6

Being a living donor

NONDIRECTED KIDNEY DONATION
KATIE AND MARK'S STORY

Katie knew very well the importance of organ donation. Her job at Mayo Clinic exposed her to it almost every day. "I knew kidney donation was extremely important from meeting patients in end-stage kidney failure, and managing the fatigue, time commitment and complications of dialysis."

Katie, a wife and mother with three young children at home, was so moved by what she saw that she decided to become a nondirected kidney donor. In nondirected donation, the donor doesn't name the specific person to get the organ. The match is arranged based on compatibility with a person in need.

"I was inspired to donate by the whole transplant and donation community, which is a community rooted in generosity and the best of medicine and surgery," Katie says. She says the evaluation experience was quite remarkable. She was, and continues to be, amazed by the dedication of all involved and how transplant teams work together across disciplines to thoroughly evaluate options for donation.

When the time came for Katie's donation, she felt well prepared and knew what to expect. Katie says her recovery was quite straightforward, and she had no problems. "I did not want to walk that first day, but with encouragement from my care team I felt better the moment I started walking around the unit. I stayed in the hospital one night, which I understand is typical. I took it easy at home for one week and was then able to return to a job that does not require physical strain. At the time of donation, our kids were 2, 4 and 6. So the key changes were not being able to pick them up for a couple of weeks, no ibuprofen and plenty of water."

Not all nondirected donors have a chance to meet their recipients, but Katie was lucky enough to do so. Her kidney went to a young woman who lived nearby. "She has become a dear friend and inspires me a great deal," Katie remarks. Since receiving Katie's kidney, the woman has started working again, has gotten engaged, and has enjoyed several adventures with her family and many four-legged friends.

Katie says she can't stress enough the importance of becoming a donor. "I deeply admire people who check the box on their license to be a donor should they have that opportunity upon their death, and those who in life donate blood, bone marrow, a kidney or a portion of their liver."

As it turns out, Katie isn't the only organ donor in her family. Her father-in-law, Mark, donated a kidney shortly after he retired as CEO for several hospitals in New York State. It's something he had been planning to do for several years. He was first inspired by his son's Eagle Scout project on organ donation and later by individuals on long-term dialysis he met during his career.

"If health is wealth, I realized my donation could extravagantly enrich another person without depleting my net worth. In fact, in some ways, I'm a richer person for having donated a kidney," says Mark. "Being part of humankind involves being kind to humans. What better way to care and share with someone else?"

And there may be more to come. Katie is considering another donation in the future. "I am hopeful to explore living liver donation as well," Katie says. After witnessing firsthand how organ donation can remarkably change a life, she feels compelled to do more.

WHO CAN BE A LIVING DONOR?

A living donor is a healthy individual who chooses to donate an organ or part of an organ — usually a kidney or part of a liver — to someone whose organ is failing. A successful transplant can help the person receiving the organ feel better, live longer, be more active and better enjoy life.

Living donors often are related to their intended recipients or are close to them in some way. This is known as directed donation. But you don't have to know the recipient to donate. If you meet the criteria, you can be a living nondirected donor.

BENEFITS TO THE RECIPIENT

Transplanting organs from living donors offers multiple advantages to recipients, such as:

- A shortened waiting time, which means that the recipient's health is likely to improve sooner. A shorter wait also reduces the risk of the recipient's health declining too much before transplant.
- Planned scheduling of the surgery, allowing for better preparation by the recipient and caregiver.
- Both surgeries can take place at the same hospital, so the organ doesn't need to travel between locations.
- Decreased risk of complications compared with deceased-donor transplants.
- The possibility of higher compatibility between living donors and candidates. In kidney transplant, this may decrease the risk of organ rejection.
- Improved odds that the organ will last longer in the recipient.

Kidney donation is the most common type of living-donor transplant. After you donate a kidney, the remaining kidney grows in size and takes on the functions of the missing kidney. You also can donate a portion of your liver. Your remaining liver regenerates rapidly and typically grows back to its original size, performing its usual functions.

Rarely, another organ, such as a lobe of a lung or a uterus, may be donated. Living donors also can donate other types of tissue for transplant, such as bone marrow and blood-forming cells, although these procedures aren't covered in this book.

Living-organ donation has increased in recent years due to the growing need for organs and a shortage of donors. Today, several thousand lifesaving living-organ donations are performed each year in the United States.

DONOR CONSIDERATIONS

Donating an organ is a big decision and shouldn't be made lightly. You should never feel pressured to donate. There are many ways to help a person who needs a transplant — you don't need to become a donor to show your support.

If you're interested in being a donor, it's important to understand what donation involves and how you feel about it. If possible, talk to someone else who has donated an organ — a family member, close friend, social worker, counselor or someone recommended by an independent donor advocate.

Questions to ask yourself before donating

Here are some questions to consider if you're thinking about donating an organ:

- How do I feel about donating? Why am I donating?
- Do I understand the medical risks?
- Are there current health concerns that might keep me from donating?
- Do I know enough about the process to make an educated decision?
- Can I afford to take the time off work to rest and recover after surgery?

- What are the long-term health and financial implications for me?
- Is someone pressuring me socially or emotionally to be a living donor?
- How will donating or not donating affect my relationship with the recipient?
- If there's more than one possible donor, how will the living donor be chosen?
- Do I have support from family members or close friends to help me through this process?
- What will my insurance cover or not cover related to the donation process?
- How will I feel if I don't meet the criteria for donation?
- Am I willing to take part in a paired donation (see page 85) if I'm not a match with the person I want to donate to?
- How will I feel if the organ I donate doesn't work well in the recipient?

These are important questions, so take your time considering them.

Requirements to be a donor
To be a donor, you must meet certain criteria. These can vary based on the type of organ you wish to donate.

Liver
Considerations related to being a liver donor include:
- **Age.** To donate a part of your liver, you must be at least 18. Most programs also will have an upper age limit of about 50 to 60 years. It takes more time for the liver to regrow as you get older. For a living liver donation to be safe for both the donor and the recipient, the liver needs to regenerate quickly.
- **Health.** You must be in good health. If you have or have had significant medical conditions, such as cancer, heart disease, lung disease or kidney disease, you may not be able to donate. Other conditions may include colon disorders, nerve problems, psychiatric disorders and other major illnesses. Sometimes a new health concern is found during the evaluation. If that happens, you may not be able to donate.

- **Blood type.** Blood type compatibility is usually required for the donor and recipient, though some programs may offer an ABO-incompatible transplant using a specific treatment protocol.
- **Your liver.** Not all livers are structured in a way that can be divided safely. Your liver must be able to be divided safely into two parts. In addition, livers vary in their configurations of blood vessels and bile ducts. The shape and size of your liver must be a good fit for the recipient. Structure and size differences are some of the most common reasons people can't donate.
- **Other health concerns.** If you smoke or drink more than a moderate amount of alcohol, you must stop before you can donate. If you carry excess weight, you may need to lose a certain amount of weight to qualify to be a living liver donor.
- **Pregnancy, birth control and hormone replacement therapy.** If you're pregnant or have recently been pregnant, you can't be a donor. In addition, it's recommended that you don't become pregnant for one year after donation. During the process of becoming a donor, you may not be able to use certain types of birth control pills, patches or injections because of clotting risks during the donation surgery. You may not be able to use hormone replacement therapy for a certain time before and after the surgery. The transplant team will provide specific guidance for you.
- **Caregivers.** All donors need caregivers to help them during recovery. Your caregiver must be a responsible adult such as a spouse, parent, sibling, adult child or friend. A caregiver should come with you to your appointments, if possible. Your caregiver and the liver transplant recipient's caregiver must be different people.
- **Follow-up care.** You must be willing to have follow-up care either at the transplant hospital or with your local healthcare team at 6, 12 and 24 months after surgery. Some people may need follow-up care beyond 24 months.

Kidney

Considerations related to being a kidney donor are similar to those involved in being a liver donor. They include:

- **Age.** You must be at least 18 years old. Some programs have a specific upper age limit, while other programs may determine if a donor is eligible on a case-by-case basis. With age, kidney function tends to decrease and risks for other health conditions increase.
- **Health.** You must be in good health. If you have significant medical conditions, you may not be able to donate. These conditions may include cancer, heart disease, liver disease and lung disease. If you've had an infectious disease that hasn't been treated, such as hepatitis or tuberculosis, you may not be able to donate until you have completed treatment.
- **Blood type.** Ideally, you and your intended recipient have a compatible blood type. If not, you may consider a paired donation. In a paired donation, your kidney is donated to someone who is compatible, and your intended recipient receives a kidney from a matched donor (see page 85). If a matched donor isn't found, then a kidney transplant where the blood types don't match may still be possible.
- **Other health concerns.** If you're a smoker or a heavy drinker, you must stop before you can donate. If you carry excess weight, you may be asked to lose weight before you donate a kidney. Along with being physically healthy, you also must be mentally and emotionally healthy.
- **Pregnancy.** If you're pregnant, you can't be a donor. If you'd like to be a kidney donor and you are thinking about becoming pregnant or have recently given birth, talk with your donor team. Often, there's a waiting period surrounding pregnancy and donation.
- **Caregivers.** All donors need caregivers to help them during recovery. Your caregiver must be a responsible adult such as a spouse, parent, sibling, adult child or friend. A caregiver should come with you to your appointments, if possible. Your caregiver and the recipient's caregiver must be different people.
- **Follow-up care.** You'll receive follow-up care with the transplant care team or with your local healthcare team. You'll need to attend follow-up visits for 4 to 6 months after surgery and again at 12 and 24 months after surgery. Some people may need follow-up care after 24 months.

Paired donation

To donate a kidney to a family member or friend, you and your intended recipient need to have compatible blood types. In addition, the transplant center conducts a crossmatch test to see if the recipient has any antibodies against your cells. A compatible blood type and a negative crossmatch mean you and your intended recipient are a good match. (See Chapter 2 for more on evaluation tests.)

If you're not a match for your intended recipient, you can still donate on behalf of your recipient through a paired donation program. A paired donation program allows for your kidney to go to someone who is a good match for it. The program then helps your intended recipient get a kidney from a different living donor. This living donor wasn't a match with their intended recipient but is a good match for your recipient. It can be complicated, so ask your transplant team to explain the process to you in detail. In some cases, paired donations may include several pairs, also called a donation chain.

The National Kidney Registry is an example of a paired donation program. Currently, there aren't any national programs that coordinate paired donations for liver transplant, although transplant centers may coordinate these types of paired donations within their own programs. For living-liver donation, the crossmatch is not an important part of determining a good match. Rather, blood type compatibility, size of the donor liver compared with the recipient and anatomy of the donor liver are important considerations.

CONSIDERATIONS

It's important to be aware of the economic considerations around organ donation. A large portion of your expenses as a living donor likely will be covered by the recipient's health insurance, but some expenses will be your responsibility. Here's what you need to consider.

Donor and recipient costs

Most medical costs related to a living donor's transplant evaluation, surgery and postoperative care are covered by the recipient's insurance.

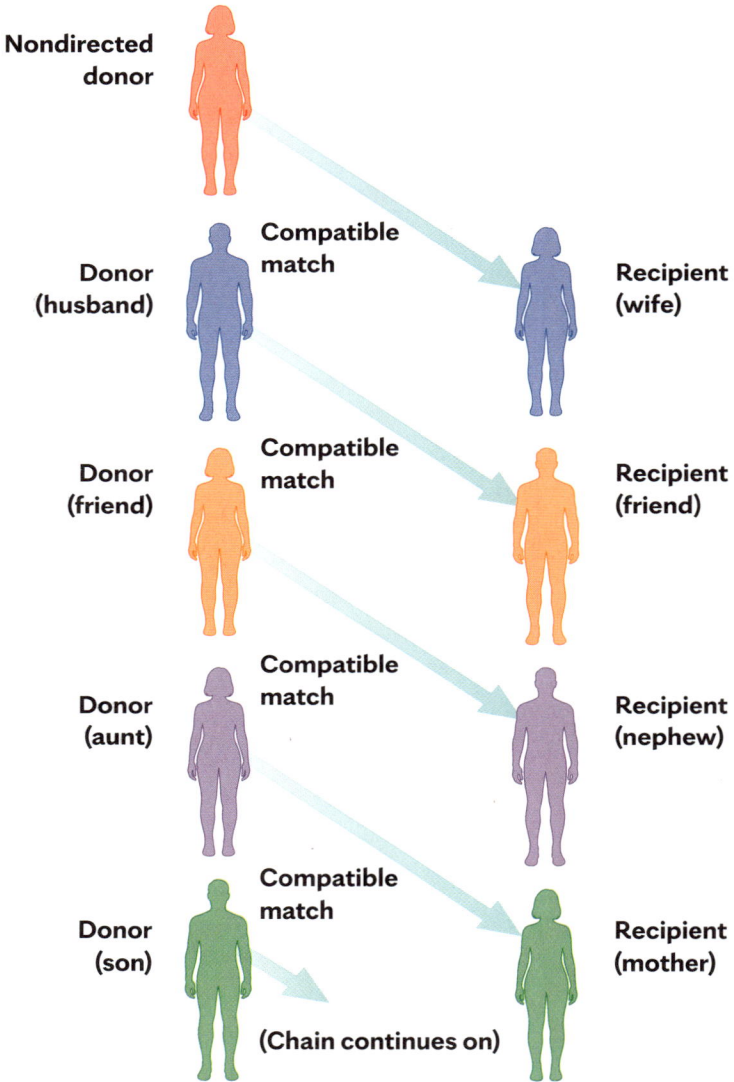

Nondirected donor

Donor (husband) — Compatible match → **Recipient (wife)**

Donor (friend) — Compatible match → **Recipient (friend)**

Donor (aunt) — Compatible match → **Recipient (nephew)**

Donor (son) — Compatible match → **Recipient (mother)**

(Chain continues on)

In an organ donation chain, more than one pair of incompatible living donors and recipients may be linked with nondirected living donors to form a donation chain in order to receive compatible organs.

Any medical issues found during the evaluation that aren't related to the donation will fall under the donor's personal health insurance coverage. For this reason, the transplant team may ask for your health insurance information before or during your evaluation. It's important to understand that any future health issues that may relate to your donation may not be covered by the recipient's insurance. Your routine medical care remains your responsibility.

Though it's uncommon, being a kidney or liver donor could affect your ability to obtain health, disability or life insurance.

Medical risks and lost work time
Donating a kidney or part of your liver means having major surgery. Some of the risks are the same as any other major surgery — infection, bleeding and blood clots. There's also a risk of complications. For example, muscle weakness at your incision site may allow a separation of the muscle after surgery and cause a bulge under your skin called an incisional hernia. Repairing it may require another surgery. Rare complications from surgery include heart attack, stroke and death.

After surgery, otherwise healthy people often feel much weaker and more tired or fatigued than they're used to feeling. The body has been through a major event. Even if everything goes as planned, it may take several weeks to months to recover fully. You'll also have a scar or scars that need to heal.

There may be days when you won't be able to do much, especially at first. It's important that you plan time for rest and recovery. For these reasons, you'll need to take time off work for surgery and recovery. Talk to your employer about the surgery. Ask about disability insurance coverage and possible paid time off. Lost wages are not covered by the recipient's insurance.

In August 2018, the U.S. Department of Labor issued an opinion letter stating that a healthy organ donor can use medical leave through the Family and Medical Leave Act (FMLA) to donate a kidney or part of a liver. Living donors whose employers offer FMLA have up to 12 weeks of unpaid, job-protected leave with their group health benefits maintained.

WORKING WITH YOUR DONOR ADVOCATE

As a living-donor candidate, you'll be assigned an independent donor advocate by the transplant center. The donor advocate is separate from the recipient's transplant team. This person represents your interests in the organ donation journey. The donor advocate makes sure that you have a good understanding of the evaluation and donation process and that you aren't being forced, coerced, pressured or financially incentivized to donate your organ.

Your donor advocate works with you throughout the donation process. If you have questions or concerns you feel uncomfortable talking about with your donor team, this person is there to help. If at any point in the process you have doubts about being a living donor, speak with your donor advocate. Remember, it's a voluntary surgery. This means you can stop the process at any point, right up to the surgery.

If you change your mind, speak to your donor advocate and alert your donor team. You don't need to give a reason or explain anything. All your discussions and decisions are confidential.

Travel and lodging

Also consider any travel and lodging expenses related to organ donation. The National Living Donor Assistance Center (see Additional resources) provides support for eligible donors' travel and lodging expenses, lost wages, and child care expenses during the evaluation and donation processes. Eligibility is determined based on a calculation of the transplant recipient's household income related to the current national poverty guidelines.

DONOR EVALUATION PROCESS

If you decide to pursue becoming a living donor, you'll go through an evaluation process. Many factors come into play for your donation to be successful, both for you and the recipient. Your donor team wants to make sure that donation is safe for you. Your team also wants to make sure that your donation will work well for the person who receives your organ.

How to apply to become a living organ donor may differ from program to program. The process typically includes a preliminary health questionnaire, phone interviews, some preliminary tests and an evaluation at the transplant center.

Health history questionnaire

The transplant program will want to know details about your current health and any past medical issues you may have experienced. You'll likely have to fill out an online health form, complete an application form or call the transplant program. Your information will go to a transplant donor coordinator or a nurse donor coordinator.

Phone interviews

The nurse donor coordinator or another transplant team member will call you within several days for a phone interview. During the interview, you'll be asked questions about yourself, your background and your medical history. You'll be informed what's involved in donating a kidney or part of your liver. A transplant social worker also may call to talk to you about organ donation. The social worker may want to verify that you're doing this voluntarily and aren't being pressured into doing it.

Blood tests

Sometimes blood tests may be required in advance of coming in for an evaluation. If so, someone with the transplant center will tell you how to obtain them.

Evaluation at the transplant center

If your blood test results are acceptable, you'll have more tests and appointments at the transplant center. These may take several days and include:

- Physical exam.
- Blood tests.

- Heart and lung function tests.
- Blood pressure tests.
- Urine tests.
- Cancer screenings.
- Imaging test, such as a chest X-ray, CT scan or MRI scan.

You'll also undergo organ-specific tests. If you're donating a kidney, you'll have a kidney function test and a detailed scan of your kidneys, bladder, and the blood vessels that carry blood to and from your kidneys. If you're donating part of your liver, you'll have similar liver-specific tests. Depending on your age and medical history, you may need additional tests.

Psychological evaluation

During your evaluation, you will meet with a transplant team member to assess your mental health. This person may be a social worker, psychologist or psychiatrist. The assessment typically involves questions about your occupation, your living arrangements and your personal life, including your engagement in certain behaviors that may impact the success of the transplant. Examples include smoking, alcohol or drug use, and factors related to the possibility of infections, including HIV, hepatitis B or hepatitis C. Team members also will want to know what kind of social support you have at home and elsewhere.

Final review

The transplant team will evaluate the information you've supplied and let you know whether you can be a living donor. The transplant team also will decide whether you're a good match for the person who may receive your donation. If you meet the necessary criteria, the team will let you know that you're eligible to donate. Transplant team members will work with you and the transplant recipient to schedule the surgery.

THE SURGERY

An advantage of living-donor surgery is that the surgery can be scheduled beforehand, allowing both the donor and the recipient to plan ahead. As a living donor, here's an idea of what you can expect during the operation. Your transplant team will give you more detailed information and instructions on how to prepare.

Liver donation surgery

Liver donation surgery usually takes about 3 to 5 hours. You and the person receiving part of your liver likely will undergo surgery at about the same time. You and the recipient will be in separate operating rooms. Both of you will have general anesthesia and be asleep during the procedures.

After making an incision in your abdomen, the surgeon will remove a part of the liver. Either the right or the left side of the liver can be used for transplant — which side is removed depends on the size of your liver and the size of the person who receives the liver. Generally, the left side of the liver is smaller than the right side. If the person you donate to is a child or a small adult, then the left side of your liver may be used. Your gallbladder also will be removed during the surgery.

The section of liver that's removed is placed in a special solution and carried to the recipient's operating room. The recipient's surgeon removes the recipient's entire liver and replaces it with your donated liver.

After the surgery, you'll likely stay in the hospital in the intermediate care or intensive care unit for a day or two. Then you'll be transferred to the transplant unit to continue your recovery. Your total stay in the hospital is likely to be 5 to 7 days.

Kidney donation surgery

Kidney donation surgery usually takes about 2 to 4 hours. Similar to liver donation surgery, you and the person receiving your kidney will undergo surgery at about the same time, but you'll be in separate operating rooms. You and the recipient will have general anesthesia, so you'll both be asleep during the operations.

During surgery, your surgeon will likely make several small incisions in your abdomen instead of one larger incision — a technique called laparoscopic surgery. Sometimes a surgeon may perform the surgery using a robotic approach. The incision sizes are similar in both robotic surgery and laparoscopy.

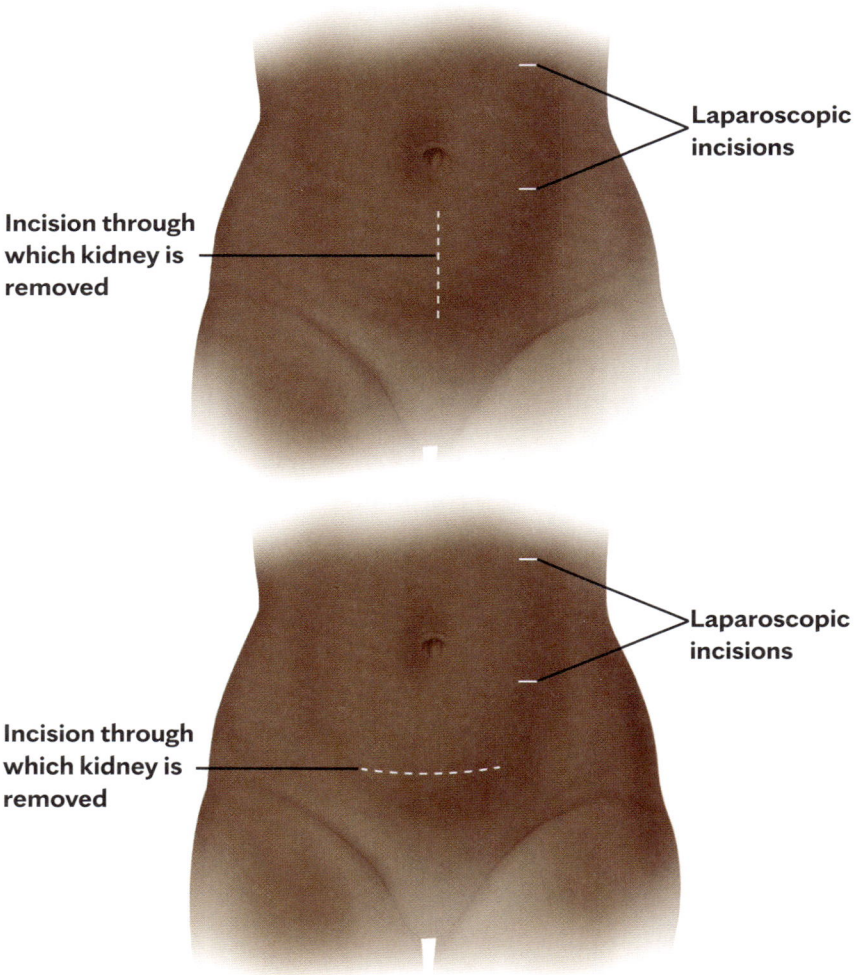

Laparoscopic incisions

Incision through which kidney is removed

Laparoscopic incisions

Incision through which kidney is removed

A surgeon typically makes one incision about 3 to 4 inches long above or below the belly button along with two laparoscopic incisions (less than 1 inch long) on the side where the kidney is removed. Surgical instruments are put through the two smaller incisions and the kidney is removed through the larger incision. Another surgeon takes that kidney and transplants it into the recipient.

After surgery, you'll likely stay in the hospital for 1 to 3 days to make sure you're recovering as expected.

AFTER SURGERY

After your surgery, it may take several weeks to start feeling more like yourself again, even after you're back home. Here are some side effects that you may experience from surgery.

Pain

Most people have some pain after surgery. Managing your pain properly can help you recover faster. Before you leave the hospital, make sure you know what pain relievers you can take. Usually, it's OK to take pain relievers that contain acetaminophen. Take the recommended dose and don't exceed it. If you have severe pain, talk to a member of your transplant team to find a pain management approach that works.

Don't take pain medicines containing aspirin or ibuprofen unless you're told you can do so. They may increase bleeding. Ask your transplant team before you take any other medicines or supplements.

Constipation

Often, surgery disrupts the gastrointestinal system. Constipation and upset stomach are common afterward. With kidney donation, your surgeon also must move your bowels to reach your kidney, which can cause your abdomen to swell and feel uncomfortable. Walking, drinking plenty of water and eating high-fiber foods can help with constipation. You also may need to use laxatives, stool softeners, suppositories or enemas for a short time. Talk to your transplant team about what's best for you.

Incision care

When you shower, gently wash your incision with mild soap. Pat it dry with a soft, clean towel. Don't put ointment, lotion or powder on your incision unless your transplant care team tells you to do so. The stitches, also called sutures, hold your incision together. They dissolve during the healing process.

Activities to avoid

To allow your body time to heal, you need to take it easy for at least a couple of months. Your transplant care team will provide specific recommendations for you. Generally, it's important for you to take the following measures:

- Don't lift anything heavier than 10 pounds for a certain period, generally at least eight weeks. Ten pounds is about as much as a gallon of milk.
- For a similar time, don't do any activities that require pushing or pulling with your upper body. For example, don't vacuum, shovel, rake or mow the lawn.
- Don't soak your incision in a bathtub, swimming pool or hot tub after surgery. This is usually for a period of 1 to 2 weeks. Showering is OK.
- Don't drive or drink alcohol until your transplant team says you may do so.
- Don't smoke for at least three months after surgery. Ideally, refrain from smoking for the rest of your life. Smoking slows the healing process.

Your healthcare team will tell you when it's safe to use certain types of birth control pills or menopausal hormone therapies after your donation. The team also can advise you on when it's safe to become pregnant. It's important to give your body enough time to fully heal.

Getting back to normal for you

After liver donation surgery, the liver begins to grow back right away. Liver regrowth is particularly rapid during the first week after surgery. It typically takes about 6 to 8 weeks for the liver to return to its original size. That's true for both the recipient and the donor. During the early part of this regrowth, you may feel more tired than usual. Most people return to work and their normal routines within 1 to 3 months, though they may still feel tired for several months.

After your kidney is removed, the other kidney increases in capacity. This phenomenon is called compensatory growth. Studies find that total kidney function returns to roughly 70% of its capacity within 10 to 11 days.

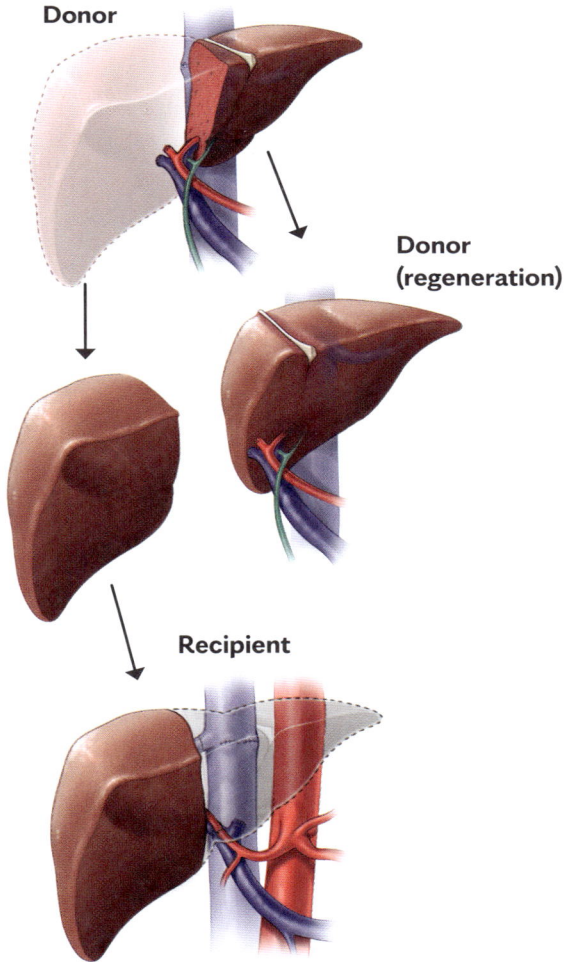

In a living-donor liver transplant, a section of liver is removed from the donor. After approximately 2 months, the donor's liver will regrow to its original size. The same growth will occur for the recipient of the donated partial liver.

Recovery from kidney donation surgery usually takes about 4 to 6 weeks. Most people return to work and their usual routines within 2 to 6 weeks depending on the type of work they do. Still, it's not unusual to feel extra tired for at least four weeks after surgery. This is because some of the usual energy you have for day-to-day activities is being used instead to help your body heal.

LIFE AFTER DONATION

Once you have fully recovered, you can generally return to your normal activities. Talk to your transplant team regarding any medication adjustments or medications to avoid after surgery. Your transplant team also will provide guidance on when it's safe to resume activities such as lifting.

General strategies for healthy living — eating a balanced diet, maintaining a healthy weight, getting enough sleep and exercising regularly — can help you to stay in good health. Additionally, you need to adhere to your follow-up appointment schedule. These appointments are usually every few months and then gradually decrease in frequency. For most people, follow-up visits continue for at least two years. Some people may need care longer than that.

The emotional aspects of your donation

It can be difficult to anticipate the emotional aftermath of your donation. You may experience several different feelings after surgery. The evaluation process and surgery can be all-consuming. Donors don't always have the opportunity to process their feelings until later. You may feel relieved that the surgery is over and happy that the recipient has a new organ.

You also may have pain. Your medications may make you feel anxious or sick. You may not sleep well in the hospital. All of this combined may make you feel worried, frustrated, irritable or sad — even while you appreciate all the effort that has gone into the organ donation.

Sometimes the transplant doesn't go as well as everyone hoped. If so, you might feel guilty or disheartened if the person you donated to is having difficulty with the new organ. And even when both the donor and the recipient are doing well, living donors sometimes still may feel depressed. These emotions are common. It's also OK to miss the part of you that you've given away, even if it sounds strange to say so. Talk to a member of your transplant team if you're dealing with strong emotions. Many living donors feel better over time.

Most donors report that giving an organ to someone in need is emotionally satisfying. Most donors go on to live active, healthy lives while seeing the positive impact of their donation on the loved one. Some say it brings them peace, joy, clarity and hope. Others say donation gives them a new perspective and makes them view themselves, their families and the world differently. Some studies find that less than 1% regret the decision. In other studies, 80% to 97% of donors say that, in retrospect, they made the right decision.

A VISIT WITH MAYO CLINIC TRANSPLANT SURGEON MIKEL PRIETO, M.D.

I'm a transplant surgeon. I also do a lot of kidney donor surgeries each year. This means I take kidneys out of perfectly healthy people . . . and give them to their loved ones, their friends or sometimes perfect strangers. I only do this because I'm confident that I'm not going to be harming the donor.

So, the first message that I tell my patients is that they'll be fine after donating a kidney. We do this typically 4 to 6 times a week. We wouldn't do it if we were harming people.

When people are thinking about being a kidney donor, they must realize that it will likely be a rewarding experience for them too. They are changing somebody's life!

Especially if they know that person well — if it's a spouse, a child or a friend that they're going to see frequently for many years. They'll see that person enjoying a full life, knowing that they had a big part in that "miracle." It's hard to match that kind of feeling. That's why it's called the gift of life.

7

While you wait

You've completed the evaluation process and you're now on a transplant waitlist. You've also gone over your financial planning and resolved your transplant questions with your insurance carrier. You've picked your transplant center and you know what lies ahead. Those are big milestones in your transplant journey. You may feel that you're all ready to go, but nothing seems to be happening. The waiting period has begun.

HOW THE WAITLIST WORKS
People waiting for the offer of a donor organ will likely tell you that it requires a lot of patience and fortitude. You hope your transplant call will come soon, but it's hard to tell when it will happen. Your transplant care team may have an estimate of how long the average wait time is at their transplant center, but everyone's wait times are different.

Wait times depend on many factors, including the urgency of your situation, how quickly you're matched with an organ donor and where you are on the transplant waitlist.

Wait times for organs also vary between different organ types. For example, most people wait 3 to 5 years for a kidney and from 1 month to 5 years for a liver. People waiting for a lung transplant typically wait several weeks to several months, while those waiting for a heart transplant may wait several days to several years.

Unlike the line at a grocery store, the transplant waitlist doesn't move sequentially. When an organ becomes available, an organ procurement organization (OPO) enters the donor's medical information into the national United Network for Organ Sharing (UNOS) computer system. The donor's information includes factors such as organ size and condition, blood type, and tissue type. The computer system generates a list of candidates compatible with the donor, taking into consideration the distance between the donor's hospital and the recipient's hospital. The OPO notifies transplant centers of potential matches, which transplant teams then consider for their patients.

The transplant team may accept or decline the organ offer, depending on whether it's the right match for the patient. If an organ is turned down for one patient, it's offered to the next person on the waitlist who's waiting for that organ. This continues until the organ is placed.

A donated organ must be preserved to stay "alive" while it travels from the donating hospital to the hospital where it will be transplanted. Different types of organs can stay preserved in cold solutions for different lengths of time. Though the organ may "live" longer, surgeons generally prefer not to have a kidney outside the body for more than 24 hours, while for the pancreas it's half that time. For the liver, preferred time outside the body is less than 8 hours, and for the heart and lungs less than 6 hours.

The introduction of various types of organ perfusion systems — through which donated organs are kept "alive" with warm, oxygenated blood or specific solutions in a specialized chamber — has allowed organs to be preserved outside the body for longer periods.

Living with so much uncertainty can be nerve-racking. It may seem as if your entire life is on hold or that you'll never get the

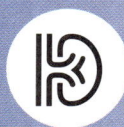

KIDNEY

→ 18 hrs.
→ 24 hrs.

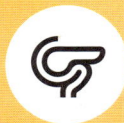

PANCREAS

→ 8 hrs.
→ 12 hrs.

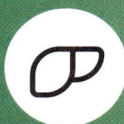

LIVER

→ 6 hrs.
→ 8 hrs.

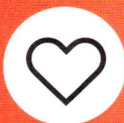

HEART/LUNGS

→ 4 hrs.
→ 6 hrs.

transplant call. You may feel that you've come so far in your transplant journey only to get stuck at the end.

You also may hear that someone who was placed on the transplant waitlist later than you has been called for a transplant procedure before you. This can be discouraging but remember that transplant is not a first-come, first-served process. If someone got a transplant sooner than you, it simply means a match was found faster.

CARING FOR YOUR PHYSICAL HEALTH

It's easy to feel frustrated, depressed and worried while you're waiting for an organ, but you can try to use this time to your advantage. Because a transplant can be a physically challenging procedure, it's helpful to go into the process as fit and well rested as possible. There's a lot that you can do to prepare yourself for a successful transplant — from exercise to nutrition and managing stress.

Move as much as you can

If you're able to exercise, regular exercise can help you stay fit, boost your energy levels and improve your mood. Being active helps lower blood sugar and blood pressure and makes you stronger. It also helps you sleep better. Even walking around your home can help.

Ask your transplant care team about the right amount of physical activity for you. Come up with a plan that works and stick to it. If you don't have the energy to exercise, your transplant care team may suggest making changes to your diet or lifestyle so you can become more active.

Eat a healthy diet

Eating nutritious foods and maintaining a healthy weight are crucial to transplant success. Maintaining a healthy weight can help reduce the chances of complications from transplant surgery and shorten the recovery time.

If you have too much weight for your body frame, your transplant care team may suggest changing your diet or increasing your physical activity. Changes to diet or physical activity can help you lose weight in preparation for your transplant.

Sometimes people waiting for a transplant struggle with getting enough nutrients to maintain good health. If you have trouble eating, your transplant team can help you take steps to improve your nutrition, such as planning meals that are tasty and easy to consume.

Pay attention to your oral health

Dental health is important. That's because dental problems can affect your recovery. Take care of any dental problems or routine procedures before your transplant. For example, bleeding gums can lead to an infection, especially when you're taking high doses of immunosuppressant medications right after the transplant.

To decrease the risk of infections after surgery, your transplant care team will ask you to postpone dental visits for a period of time after the surgery. This is usually for at least the first four months after transplant.

Stay current on vaccinations

Ask your transplant care team what vaccines you may need. Immuno-suppressant medications — required after transplant to prevent rejection — dampen your immune response to vaccines. So it's best to get all your recommended vaccinations before transplant surgery.

Get enough sleep

Sleep plays a major role in maintaining your physical and mental health and building your resilience. Getting enough sleep helps reduce stress, depression and anxiety. It also helps maintain energy levels and a positive mood.

An ideal amount of sleep is 7 to 9 hours daily. Establish a regular sleep schedule and routine such as going to bed at the same time every day. Practice good sleep hygiene — unplug from electronics, read a book, dim your lights and set aside your worries for the night.

Stay away from tobacco and alcohol

If you haven't stopped smoking or drinking alcohol already, you need to do so in order to safely undergo transplant surgery. Smoking can interfere with healing and increase the risk of transplant complications, including infection, blood clotting, organ rejection and cancer. Alcohol isn't healthy for the liver and is associated with several health conditions. If you need help quitting smoking or drinking alcohol, ask your transplant care team for advice.

CARING FOR YOUR MENTAL WELL-BEING

Learning how to cope with difficult, sometimes big emotions and to maintain a positive, resilient attitude is a critical part of your transplant journey. It's also important to the success of your treatment. Active coping — having a plan for managing stressful events — is linked to better quality of life in transplant patients.

Dealing with difficult emotions

While going through your transplant journey, you may experience a range of complex emotions. You may be reflecting on your past or feel anxious about the future. You also may feel that your illness has taken away your ability to enjoy life. Here are some difficult emotions that you may be dealing with — and some suggestions for how to overcome them.

Fear

It's difficult to wait for a lifesaving treatment. People waiting for a transplant are often afraid that they won't make it to the actual procedure. This is a common feeling, but train your thoughts and intentions toward the following:

- Believe that your transplant care team is doing everything possible to make sure you receive a transplant in a timely manner.
- Carefully follow all the instructions your transplant care team gave you to keep your condition stable until the transplant happens.
- Take your medications exactly as prescribed, especially as this relates to pain management.

Worry and sadness

Dealing with a chronic condition and going through the transplant process can be arduous, stressful and full of uncertainty, and may lead you to experiencing feelings of worry and sadness.

If you have these feelings, try to focus on moments of joy. Celebrate happy occasions with your family and friends. Find reasons to laugh and engage in activities you enjoy. Take good care of yourself, including moving as much as you can, spending time in nature, getting enough sleep and eating nutritious foods.

If you have ongoing anxiety or sadness that won't go away, talk to your care team about finding professional help. Taking care of your mental health is an important part of your treatment plan.

Grief

Many people on a transplant list experience grief or a sense of loss. For example, you may feel that you've lost part of your identity because you need a transplant. You may feel that you've lost opportunities or dreams for your future or that you've lost control of your life. You may grieve over how your health has affected personal relationships or your career.

Acknowledging these losses is part of your path to recovery. At the same time, try to reflect on the progress you've made so far and how it may have stretched your identity in new, perhaps even more fulfilling, directions. Focus on relationships that nurture and support you. If you can accept what's happening with your life, it may allow you to set new goals for your future.

Guilt

People waiting for an organ sometimes feel guilty, thinking that others must die for them to live. But this thinking is not accurate. Donors don't die so that others can live. They die because no one is immortal. Upon a donor's death, the family is following the donor's wishes to donate the organs to save lives. Or the family is making a decision on behalf of their loved one because they know it's something their loved one would have wanted.

For families, being able to honor the wishes of their loved ones and also provide a lifesaving gift for waiting recipients can sometimes provide some comfort.

There are ways for a recipient to thank the donor's family, and many recipients find it helpful to do so (see pages 230-231).

Regret

Some people waiting for a transplant feel regret for various reasons. Instead, focus on the future, which you can shape. Look at your transplant journey as a fresh chapter in your life that can provide new meaning and purpose.

Being a burden

Donor recipients sometimes feel that they've become a burden to those around them. In a typical household, for example, couples often split their responsibilities. One spouse may cook while the other mows the lawn. A chronic illness may take away a person's ability to fulfill previous roles, transferring those responsibilities to other family members, who also may become caregivers.

You didn't choose to become ill — it happened. Your job now is to progress through your transplant milestones so that you'll be ready for the procedure when it comes. Many transplant recipients say that the time when they were dependent on their loved ones was precious. As you go through your transplant journey with your caregiver, your relationship may grow and blossom in ways you couldn't imagine.

The best way to help yourself right now may be to lean on others for the assistance you need without feeling bad about it. It's OK to ask your family and friends to mow the lawn, shovel the driveway, walk the dog, cook dinner or pick up your kids. You'd do the same for them if they were in a challenging life situation. Likewise, most people will want to help you.

How to improve your well-being

A key step to staying resilient while on the transplant waitlist is to find tools that address the health of your whole person — mind, body and spirit. Here are some strategies that may be helpful.

- **Exercise.** Regular exercise helps increase your physical fitness, flexibility and stamina. It improves mood, increases energy levels, and stimulates your immune system and metabolism. It also can help regulate weight. All of this is important for getting you ready for your transplant.
- **Meditation.** Meditation can bring you relaxation, calmness, mental clarity and emotional balance. The practice can take many forms, including being mindful of the present moment, focusing your thoughts on favorite sights or smells, and praying.
- **Tai chi.** Sometimes described as meditation in motion, this series of movements is performed in a slow, graceful manner. Tai chi can help you reduce stress and improve balance, stamina and energy.
- **Biofeedback.** You can use a variety of monitoring devices, including devices that measure heart rate, skin temperature and brain activity, to moderate certain body responses. These responses include blood pressure, heart rate and muscle tension. If you're interested, ask your healthcare team or transplant care team.
- **Progressive muscle relaxation.** To practice this relaxation technique, you work your way through your body from head to toe,

CHOOSING A SUPPORT GROUP THAT'S RIGHT FOR YOU

There are several kinds of support groups for people on a transplant list. Think about whether one of these might be helpful to you.

Hospital groups

Hospital groups are usually run by the hospital transplant coordinator, social worker or other member of the transplant team.

- Typically consists of patients who are either waiting for a transplant or recovering after transplant.
- Usually meets more frequently than groups not connected to the hospital.

Local support groups

Local support groups are typically run by transplant patients or their family members. They help people who have already had their transplants adjust to their new lives and help others do the same. Support groups also can help people still on the waitlist keep their spirits high.

- Usually consists of patients waiting for a transplant and recovering after a transplant, as well as their families.
- Typically have monthly meetings and special events.

Online support groups

You can find many groups on Facebook and other social media websites that focus on a particular organ type, such as kidney, liver or heart. Use your good judgment about online support groups. Make sure you're comfortable with the group and the information that you're receiving.

- Generally consists of people with a range of transplant experiences. Participants may come from all over the world.
- You can ask personal questions in the comfort of your own home and at any time of the day or month.

tightening and releasing each muscle group as you go. As you let the muscle tension go, you may be able to release feelings of anxiety or stress from your mind too.

Keep in mind that not all activities may be right for you. What is right for you depends on your specific health situation. Talk to your transplant care team about what might work best for your situation.

If you feel that despite your best efforts, your mental health is worsening, you're losing interest in life, you can't sleep or you have suicidal thoughts, alert your care team right away. Treatment, such as counseling or medications, can help you achieve a better mental state, and that can help you be better prepared for the transplant procedure and your life afterward.

STAYING ORGANIZED

There's a lot going on, even while you're waiting. Having a system that makes key daily tasks easy to complete and keeps important information at your fingertips can be very helpful now and in the future. Here are some recommended strategies for people on a transplant waitlist.

Keep track of appointments and medications

You'll continue to meet with your transplant team while you're on the waitlist. This is needed so that your care team can monitor your health and periodically reassess your risks and the urgency of your situation. A paper notebook or digital planner can help you keep track of all your appointments, test procedures and results. It also can help you stay on top of your medication schedules.

Stay focused

Follow your transplant care team's treatment plan carefully. Take your medications as instructed and stick to the exercise routine your transplant care team recommended. Practice healthy-lifestyle habits such as avoiding smoking and drinking alcohol. If you're on dialysis, don't miss your dialysis sessions. Focus on staying in the best shape possible to make your recovery faster and easier.

TALKING TO FAMILY AND FRIENDS ABOUT LIVING ORGAN DONATION

If you're waiting for a kidney or liver transplant and you're running out of time to receive one from a deceased donor, you might consider looking for a living donor. A living donor is someone who's willing to donate a kidney or a portion of a liver. These donations are possible because a person can live with just one kidney and the liver can regenerate to its original size.

Many people may not know that they can help save a loved one with such a donation and still maintain a good quality of life. Consider talking to family members and friends about how living donation works and how it may save your life.

Certainly, asking someone to donate an organ or a part of an organ to you can be awkward or challenging. Try talking to your family and friends about such a donation without asking for anything. Share some information about your health situation and how you may not get the transplant in time. For example, if you're waiting for a kidney transplant, you may say something like this:

> The results of my recent medical tests confirm that my kidneys are failing. As my kidney function gets worse, my options will be dialysis or a transplant. Dialysis is an artificial way of filtering my blood through a machine. This typically takes a few hours and occurs three days a week. Over time, dialysis can be hard on a person's health. A kidney transplant typically provides a better quality of life over the long term.

> The number of people waiting for a kidney transplant from a deceased donor is much greater than the number of available organs. And the longer I'm on dialysis, the greater my risk of complications becomes. The sicker I am, the more difficult it will be to get through and recover from transplant surgery.

Another way I could get a transplant before I get very sick is from a living donor. A healthy person can give me a kidney because people need just one healthy kidney. With a living donor, I can receive a transplant sooner. Plus, kidney transplants from living donors often last longer and work better than do donated kidneys from people who have died.

As you share this information with family and friends, they're likely to have questions. For example, they may ask:

- What are the risks to the donor?
- What medical tests does the donor need?
- How long is the surgery and recovery?
- Can anyone donate a kidney? Who is the ideal donor?
- Will the donor have to pay for the surgery?

You can find more information about what's involved in living organ donation in Chapter 6. If family and friends are interested in learning more, connect them to your transplant care team. If one of them is found to be a good match, your transplant wait time may be quicker than you expected.

The popularity of living-organ donation has increased dramatically in recent years due to the growing need for organs for transplantation and the shortage of available organs from deceased donors. Living-donor organ transplants also tend to result in fewer complications than deceased-donor organ transplants and, overall, longer survival of the donor organ.

Take notes

Carry a notebook or smartphone with you to all appointments and take notes. Keep a running list of questions for your transplant team. Prepare a phone and email contact list to update your family and friends when your transplant time comes. This also will make it easier for your caregiver to keep your loved ones up to date while you're going through surgery and recovery.

Make necessary arrangements

If you have young children, have a child care plan in place for the time you'll be away. If you have pets, arrange for pet care. Ask your transplant care team when you might expect to see your children and pets after your transplant. If you need to take an extended sick leave from your job, now may be the right time to fill out the paperwork. Organize your personal information — for example, share access to your bank accounts, email account or phone apps with a trusted family member or friend.

Keep learning

Learn as much as possible about your transplant procedure, the medications you'll need to take and the recovery process. Learn the relevant medical terminology. The transplant process comes with a language of its own, full of medical terms, abbreviations and acronyms. The more "medical speak" you understand, the better you'll be able to navigate through your transplant journey.

Plan ahead

Visit the transplant center. Ask for a walk-through and information about what to expect when you receive the call. This may help lessen your stress. And it may help you better prepare and be more familiar with your surroundings when you arrive for your transplant surgery.

Make travel and relocation arrangements

Arrange your transportation for the moment when your transplant call comes. You'll have to get to the transplant center quickly when an organ becomes available. For example, you may want to plan the driving route and think about traffic conditions. If you're relocating closer to your hospital, make housing arrangements and focus on settling in at your home away from home.

Start a bag

You also may want to keep a bag that is packed and ready to go so that you're not scrambling at the last minute. You'll need to be ready to leave as soon as you get the call. Having your bag packed in advance can save time. Make sure to include your insurance information, the list of medications you're taking, an extra 24-hour supply of medications, phone chargers, glasses or contact lenses if you use them, and other necessities.

Keep your phone on

Always answer your phone! When you get an offer, you'll need to be at the hospital within a short window of time. Be ready for medical tests and possibly a long wait for surgery.

FOR CAREGIVERS: KEY CAREGIVER ROLES

Waiting for a transplant call can be taxing on caregivers too. You may feel that your life is also on pause and you aren't able to make any future plans of your own. You may feel anxious and restless and stuck. But similar to the person in your care, you can use the waiting time to better prepare for what lies ahead. When the transplant call comes, you want to be as prepared as possible. You'll be the person in charge from that point on. Remember, without you, your loved one can't successfully complete the transplant journey.

Be organized

Partner with the person in your care to keep track of appointments and medication schedules. People waiting for a transplant often experience poor health, which may affect their ability to focus and remember things. They may forget about a test procedure or miss a dose of medication. They may need help understanding the next steps. You may need to keep track of your loved one's medications and procedures.

CAREGIVER CHECKLIST

- ☐ Stay in communication with the person getting the transplant.
- ☐ Go to appointments.
- ☐ Help communicate changes.
- ☐ Prepare a travel or relocation plan.
- ☐ Try to maintain your normal lifestyle.
- ☐ Find support resources.

Communicate regularly

Keep checklists, take notes, and write down questions. Stay in touch with the transplant care team. Provide the team with regular updates on how the person in your care is doing. If health changes happen, your loved one may need to undergo more tests. And the transplant care team may determine that the need for a transplant is more urgent, which can shorten your loved one's wait time.

Become an expert

Use this time to learn as much as possible to understand what lies ahead for you. Take a caregiver education class at your transplant center. Subscribe to email newsletters from your transplant center and transplant organizations such as UNOS to stay up to date. Find foundations and nonprofit organizations that focus on the type of transplant your loved one is waiting for and join their email lists. These organizations may offer educational events and webinars as well as support groups.

Build support networks

Find and join transplant support groups or ask the transplant social worker for suggestions. (See page 116 for more on the different types of support groups.) You also may want to join a caregiver support group, which focuses specifically on aspects of the caregiver's journey.

You may find it helpful to connect with people who are going through similar experiences, so you can share tips and other useful information. You may want to ask questions of other caregivers with loved ones who are already recovering from surgery. For example, you can ask how best to prepare for surgery and what to expect during recovery. Share your concerns and questions with them. You may make new friends who understand what you're going through better than anyone else.

Take care of yourself
If you're relocating to be closer to the hospital, you may feel over-whelmed and stressed about moving and settling in a new place. Find ways to relax, such as practicing yoga, meditation, deep breathing or tai chi. Stay active, exercise, and eat nutritious foods so that you have enough energy for your loved one's transplant journey. Remember that you'll need all your physical and mental strength at the time of transplant and during recovery.

8

Waiting with your child

Having a child on the organ transplant waitlist can feel like your world has been turned upside down. This time will undoubtedly bring a roller coaster of emotions.

The uncertainty of when the call will come and the need to always be ready for it can be very stressful. Before surgery, you may feel overwhelmed by all the little details that need to be taken care of. And what about the transplant itself? Will it be successful?

Feeling anxious about how things will go for your child is completely understandable. People may tell you how strong your family is during this journey. But you might feel quite the opposite, considering it more like a challenge that you didn't ask for and one you're struggling to get through. These emotions are valid, and it's OK not to feel very strong.

But then there are those feelings that keep you going — hope and optimism that the call will come soon, the surgery will be successful, and a healthier childhood is within reach. There are feelings of gratitude that someone is generous enough to donate an organ — though it's common also to feel sadness that another family is undergoing a tragedy.

Whatever you may be feeling right now, know that others in your position have experienced similar emotions. And know that your child's transplant team has helped other families navigate this difficult time. Don't hesitate to lean on the team. In the meantime, getting things in order so that you're ready can help you feel like you have some control over your life and all that is happening.

PREPARING FOR THE CALL

The organ transplant waitlist is a national database that lists everyone waiting for a transplant. At any given time, more than 100,000 people are awaiting an organ match. Of these, more than 2,000 are under the age of 18. While that can sound intimidating, it's not the same as waiting in line at the grocery store.

The waitlist is a pool of potential organ recipients. When an organ becomes available, the first call goes to the person who is the best match to the donor. So, it's not first come, first served. Unless your child is undergoing a living-donor transplant for a kidney or liver, it's hard to know when the match will occur, though your team should be able to provide some guidance.

With that in mind, here are some steps you can take to make sure you're ready.

Prioritize good health

While it's important to try to keep life as normal as possible, it's also very important to keep your child as healthy as you can while you wait for a transplant. Some children may be in the hospital during this time; other children may be at home. Here's what you can do:

- Make sure your child attends all appointments and follows the treatment plan mapped out by the transplant team. All medicines should be taken in the correct dose and at scheduled times. Now is an excellent time to check that your child is up to date on vaccines. Check that anyone who interacts regularly with your child is up to date on vaccines too. The transplant team can advise you on which vaccines your child should have.

With so many factors involved in matching organ donors to organ recipients, there's no way to know when a call will come. Sometimes, an organ is found relatively quickly. Other times, it takes several years. The goal is to find your child the best match possible to minimize the risk of complications and offer your child the best chance at a healthy life moving forward.

Given your child's specific health needs and organ availability in the area where the medical center is located, your transplant care team can offer you tailored insight on a realistic wait time. Typical factors influencing the wait time for an organ include:

- **Organ type.** The organ needed significantly impacts wait times. Kidneys, livers, hearts, lungs and other organs have different availability rates. For some organs, such as kidneys, being under the age of 18 moves you up higher on the list.
- **Blood type and tissue match.** Compatibility between the donor and recipient is crucial. Blood type and tissue matching ensure that the recipient's body is less likely to reject the organ. Some blood types are more common, making it easier to find a match.
- **Medical urgency.** The severity of a child's condition plays a role. Children in critical condition may be prioritized higher on the list to receive an organ.
- **Geographical location.** Availability can vary by region. Some areas have more donors relative to patients, leading to shorter wait times, while other areas may have a longer list of recipients.

- Follow any specific dietary restrictions or guidelines provided by the transplant team.
- Encourage good hygiene, such as hand-washing before eating and after every bathroom visit. Try to avoid being around people who are sick, and have your child wear a mask when appropriate.

Organs also can only live outside the body for a short time, so how fast you can get to a transplant center matters (see page 110).

- **Size and age.** For hearts, lungs and livers, the size of the donor and recipient must be similar. In certain liver transplantations, it may be possible to separate the liver into two separate sections called lobes.
- **Time on the waitlist.** In some cases, the length of time a child has been on the waitlist moves the child closer to the top of the list. In other cases, as mentioned earlier, priority is given to children with more severe illness. For a child awaiting a kidney transplant, the child's waitlist position also includes any time spent on dialysis.

Some families do multilisting, which means a child is listed at more than one transplant center. Listing at multiple centers may increase your child's chances of getting an organ more quickly, as you'll have access to a larger donor pool.

However, there are a few things to consider with multiple listings. You'll need to meet in person with each transplant center that your child is listed with. You'll also need to make it to the transplant center within the time period recommended by the transplant team if an organ becomes available there. You also want to make sure that your insurance provider will cover the cost of multiple-site testing. Check with your transplant care team to see if there's a benefit to adding your child to multiple centers.

Be honest and open with your child

Your child likely will have many questions during this waiting period. Be honest and try giving answers in a way that is easy to understand. For younger children who are asking why they need a new organ, simply explain that their organ is no longer working correctly, and it needs to be replaced. For children nervous that they're the only ones going through this, reassure them that there are other children who also need new organs. Encourage your child to express feelings and ask questions. This can help your child feel more in control and less anxious.

Even if your child isn't asking many questions, make sure your child understands what will happen. Children have great imaginations! Consider asking your child to describe what having surgery will mean so you can clear up any misconceptions your child may have.

This is also a good time to enlist the help of a child life specialist, if one is available on your child's transplant team. This person is trained to explain the transplant process to children and help them deal with the complex feelings they may be experiencing.

You can help maintain a sense of normalcy by allowing your child to take part in regular activities and play as long as it's safe. Some children are very sick as they await a transplant and may spend this time waiting in the hospital. Talk to your child's care team to ensure your child remains engaged in age-appropriate activities.

Be reachable

Make sure your child's transplant care team has all of your contact information. It's also helpful to provide emergency contacts in case you're not reachable for any reason.

Always have your phone with you and ringer turned on so you don't miss a call from the transplant center. This call may include detailed instructions from the transplant care team on the next steps. Consider keeping pen and paper handy to write down all the instructions when you get the call, such as when to have your child stop eating and drinking in preparation for surgery and which medicines or other treatments to stop.

Stay organized

It's easy — and understandable — to feel overwhelmed when your child is facing a transplant. To help you stay organized, try using a smartphone app or keep a binder of all your child's medical records and appointments and any notes you take during those appointments.

This goes for non-medical-related tasks too. You may find it helpful to use calendars or other reminders to pay monthly household expenses, such as utilities, rent or mortgages.

Plan ahead

To start, pack the essentials. You'll need insurance cards, medicines and clothing for you and your child, as well as other items, such as your child's favorite blanket or stuffed animal, to make a hospital stay comfortable. Then:

- Talk to loved ones about stepping in on a moment's notice to look after your other children or to care for your pets in your absence. You may want to appoint someone close to you to be the go-to person for updating family and friends when you no longer can.
- Plan your route to the transplant center or airport. Look at alternative routes in case of heavy traffic, an accident or construction.
- Plan where you'll stay during and after the transplant. The transplant team's social worker should be able to provide you with a list of options.
- Take note of what to do when you get to the transplant center. Ask the social worker or another team member where to go once you get there, where to park, how visiting hours work and other rules.

Some of these details might seem small, but having a comprehensive plan can help your family be prepared and ready to go when you get the call.

Create a support network

Consider connecting with other parents in the same situation. Often, they can be your best emotional support resources. Talk with your transplant center's social worker about available support groups. If there aren't other parents in your area with similar experiences, online social media communities and sites such as United Network for Organ Sharing (UNOS) can help fill the gaps.

Financial planning

Your transplant center's financial counselor can help you understand the costs involved and explore options for financial assistance. Depending on where you live, your child may be eligible for Medicaid or the Children's Health Insurance Program (CHIP).

Organizations such as the Children's Organ Transplant Association provide financial support to families in need. Fundraising and applying for grants also can help cover expenses. However, money raised through sources such as crowd-funding sites can sometimes incur taxes and impact state program eligibility. Your transplant team's financial coordinator can help guide you.

If you need to take time off from work, meet with someone from your employer's human resources department well in advance. The Family and Medical Leave Act (FMLA) helps protect your job while you're away. In some states, you also may be entitled to paid time off to help care for your child.

Address potential obstacles

The reality is, for some children on the waitlist, an organ might never come, or their condition may deteriorate and make transplant impossible. Talk with the transplant team about what other treatment options may be available for your child.

Sometimes, you might have to deal with unexpected setbacks. Your child may develop an infection that makes it too risky to undergo surgery. If so, your child may be moved from "active" status on the waitlist to "inactive" — meaning matches won't be considered until your child's health improves. This can be frustrating and disappointing. Discuss with the transplant team in advance how these situations are handled.

Practice self-care

Waiting for your child's transplant is like running a marathon. You, as the caregiver, need to be in good shape in preparation for the journey ahead. Exercise when you can, eat well, get enough sleep, and consider mindfulness techniques such as meditation or yoga to keep yourself in good health. Seek counseling if you need additional support. Remember, caring for yourself is vital so you can fully be there for your child.

IT'S A MATCH

As you read earlier, the transplant waitlist is a national database overseen by the Organ Procurement and Transplantation Network (OPTN).

COPING WITH A DRY RUN

There are times when a family will accept an offer and head to the transplant center, only to learn through test results that the organ isn't a good match after all. You can read more about this on page 138.

Being told at this point that the transplant can't happen can be very disappointing and may create feelings of anger, grief, fear and a host of other strong emotions. Know that the transplant team's core mission is to make sure your child has the best transplant outcome possible. A less-than-ideal match or an organ that's not as healthy as expected can create many problems after transplant, including organ rejection.

Trust the members of your transplant care team if they determine the match doesn't meet their standards and lean on them for support.

Organ procurement organizations (OPOs) manage organ donations and recoveries. And the United Network for Organ Sharing (UNOS), a nonprofit organization, runs the computer system that matches recipients with donors. For more information on these organizations, see the Additional resources section at the end of the book.

When someone dies and an organ is donated, an organ procurement organization enters information about the organ's size, condition, blood type and tissue type into the database. The computer system, which runs continuously, generates a list of potential candidates from the waitlist who closely match the donor's characteristics.

If your child is a good match, your transplant center will be notified that an organ is available. This is called an offer. The transplant team will discuss whether this is the best match, often deciding in a matter of minutes. A transplant team may turn down an offer if the team doesn't think the organ is a good match. In these cases, the organ will be offered to the next person on the list.

If the organ is a good match, the transplant team will call you and ask whether you accept the offer. If you do, the process of getting the organ to the transplant center begins. The transplant team also may notify you that your child is a backup for an organ. This is when an organ is available for someone else, but if that person can't receive it, your child will receive the offer instead.

In most cases, you'll have only minutes to decide whether to accept the organ. It's not unusual to panic or think your child or your family isn't ready for the offer. If you're feeling scared or unsure, or if there's anything that's preventing you from accepting the offer, address your questions to your transplant team. The team can provide answers and offer reassurance. It's important to remember that your transplant team won't offer your child an organ unless it's a good match for your child.

When you get to the hospital, it's likely that your child will go through additional testing to prepare for surgery. This includes a round of testing designed to confirm that the organ is a good match. Sometimes, the organ is not a good match.

If your child is confirmed to be a good match, your child will proceed to the next steps in preparation for surgery. For more on what to expect during transplant surgery, see Chapter 12.

9

Pack your bags

You might be eating breakfast, cleaning up after dinner or walking your dog. Perhaps you're watching a nightly television show before turning out the lights and drifting off to sleep. Or it could be a holiday when you're having dinner with family. Suddenly, your phone rings, and when you answer, it's someone from your transplant team informing you that they found you a match. Depending on how the notification process is set up at your transplant center, the person calling could be a transplant coordinator, a transplant nurse or your surgeon.

While you're waiting for a transplant, it's important to answer your phone at all times of day and night so that you don't miss an offer from your transplant center. Many transplant centers will ask you to identify a backup person for them to call who may be able to reach you in case the transplant center is not able to.

When you finally get that call, you may feel a surge of adrenaline, excitement or eagerness. You might experience a peaceful state of being ready and happy it's going to happen. You also may feel anxious and nervous. Some people may be frightened about the surgery or sad for the family that lost a loved one, but at the same moment they're thrilled to receive their gift. All of these feelings are normal.

You also may feel that the phone call is the finish line you've been waiting to cross. In reality, it's just the beginning of a new step in your transplant journey.

THE CALL

When you get a call with an organ offer from your transplant center, a member of the transplant care team typically asks you a few questions and then shares some important information. You want to listen carefully and take notes because the instructions may be complex.

After informing you about the match, you may be asked questions about your current health and your overall readiness for transplant. These questions typically include:

- Have you had any changes in your health?
- Have you had any recent infections or hospitalizations?
- Have you had any recent blood transfusions?
- Are you able to get to the transplant center right now?
- Is your caregiver able to come with you?
- Do you have transportation to get to the hospital?
- Are there any insurance changes?

The caller also may share some information about the organ being donated. This won't include any personal data related to the donor, but you'll learn important health-related information, such as any potential risks related to the organ being offered.

For example, your donor may test positive for certain viruses often found in humans, such as the Epstein-Barr virus, cytomegalovirus, herpes or other viruses. These are generally considered manageable and usually are easy to treat. Some donors may test positive for hepatitis A, B or C. Depending on your situation, these findings may not be showstoppers either because modern medicines can effectively treat these conditions.

The conversation with the caller is intended to help you make an educated choice about the offer. At the end, you'll be asked to give your verbal consent to proceed with the surgery. It's important to know that your transplant team will never suggest moving ahead with an organ that the team doesn't think is good for you. However, if you have doubts or questions, this is the moment to ask them. You also can ask for a few minutes to think the offer over, but time is limited.

You can decide to decline the transplant offer. Declining doesn't mean that you'll be taken off the waiting list or moved to the bottom of the list. You'll return to the same spot on the transplant waiting list where you were before you got the call. Declining a transplant means that you'll go back to waiting for the next available organ. You don't "miss your spot in line." However, you won't know how soon you'll get the next offer, whether that organ will have higher or lower risks, or whether you'll remain healthy enough to receive a transplant before the next offer comes.

Accepting the offer
If you decide to accept the offer, you'll give your transplant team a verbal consent to move ahead. After that, one of two things will happen.
- You'll be told to come to the transplant center right away.
- You'll be told to remain at your residence and stand by.

If you're told to come to the hospital, your caller will tell you where to go and what time to arrive. The time you're given depends on when the organ for your transplant is expected to get there and on the type of transplant you're receiving. For example, kidneys are viable outside the body longer than hearts. So if you're getting a kidney transplant, you'll have more time to get there, but less so for a heart (see page 109). Your transplant care team also might tell you to stop eating and drinking at a specific time in preparation for the surgery.

You and your caregiver likely will have your bags packed and ready to go. Still, it's a good idea to give everything one last check (see pages 141-142). If you have time, you may want to take a quick shower. If you don't have time, don't worry about it. The most important thing is to get to the transplant center on time. Follow your transportation plan. If you're flying, depart on the earliest plane you can get tickets for.

If you're told to be on standby, be ready to travel at a moment's notice. Most often the reason you may be placed on standby is that your organ isn't ready yet. As you're waiting, many things are happening behind the scenes involving your transplant team and the organ you'll be receiving.

BEHIND THE SCENES

Before your phone rings with the transplant offer, a few things must happen first. Your surgeon or another member of the transplant team receives an organ offer that's a match for you and the donor's medical info.

A match means that the donor or family members have agreed to donate the organ once the donor passes. At the time of your call, your donor likely is still on life support and will remain on life support until the organ procurement team arrives to recover the organ.

Depending on your transplant center, the person traveling to procure your organ may or may not be your transplant surgeon. Organ donation and the recovery of donated organs are highly coordinated work. Due to the need for coordination, occasionally delays can happen that may hold up your surgery.

What happens during organ procurement

Once your procurement team arrives at the donor's hospital, team members begin the surgical process of recovering the donor's organ or organs. As they do that, they'll also assess the organ's condition. If necessary, they'll do laboratory tests to make sure it's healthy. If the organ is considered healthy enough to be transplanted, the transplant team will remove the organ from the donor and prepare it for transportation.

In the past, organs to be transplanted were flushed with a chilled preservation solution and kept cold during travel. The cold environment essentially makes the organ's cells "go to sleep" so they don't die or get damaged. The solution also has electrolytes and nutrients to nourish and sustain the organs during travel.

Today, recovered organs may be attached to devices that pump either blood or a nourishing solution through the organ's blood vessels during transportation (see pages 80-81). This process is called organ perfusion. The organ perfusion devices allow the organ to be safely outside the body for more time. They also allow surgeons to assess the organ's health more efficiently.

Once your transplant team has the organ ready to transport, the team heads back to the transplant hospital. If you're waiting on standby, you'll get another phone call telling you to come to the hospital.

What happens at the transplant hospital

When you arrive at the hospital where your surgery will happen, you likely will check in at the general admission center. You may be directed to a nursing floor or directly to the preoperative unit. Your caregiver should be able to stay with you until you're ready to go into surgery.

In the hospital, you'll meet with your surgical team. You'll speak with your surgeon and your anesthesiologist, who will explain what they're going to do. You'll go through a series of tests to ensure your health hasn't changed since your last appointment and confirm that you're still fit to undergo the surgery. The transplant care team will check your blood pressure, pulse and temperature, and run blood tests. They may do a chest X-ray and an electrocardiogram (ECG or EKG) to check your heart. You'll also sign a consent form to undergo the surgery.

As you receive your presurgical wellness check, the donated organ may undergo its own tests. The transplant team will do one last check of the organ's health. They'll look at how the organ withstood transportation. If the organ is connected to a perfusion pump, they'll check the organ's function. The pump gathers the organ's vital information frequently or continuously, similar to how a patient is monitored in an intensive care unit. If necessary, the organ can stay connected to the pump for several hours, until the team is sure it's fit for transplantation.

While this is happening, you and your caregiver may need to wait until everything is ready for the surgery. During this time, you won't be able to eat or drink — it's important to keep your stomach empty before anesthesia. Once both you and the organ pass all the checks, you'll be taken into the operating room.

How you pack for the next phase of your transplant journey depends on whether you're going to a hospital near your home or traveling to a transplant center that's far away.

When packing for a transplant operation and recovery, it's helpful to think about what you'll need in the hospital before and immediately after surgery versus what you'll need once you're discharged. Some of these items may overlap, but they aren't exactly the same. So you might want to create two different packing lists. Also consider where you'll be staying the first few weeks after the surgery. If the hospital is far from your home and you'll be staying in a temporary residence or transplant housing during recovery, you'll likely need to pack more items.

When checking in to the hospital for your surgery, bring the minimum number of items with you. Include essentials such as medicines you may need while waiting, eyeglasses, hearing aids, phone and charger, a change of clothes, and other needed items.

For example, you don't need to bring a blood pressure monitor or a thermometer with you, as hospital staff will be monitoring your vital signs. You won't need too many clothes because you'll be

When it's a dry run

In some situations, an offer doesn't result in transplantation. People may get the standby call, but they won't be asked to come to the hospital. In other cases, they may come to the hospital, only to be discharged a few hours later without the transplant. These situations are called dry runs, and they can be very upsetting. There are different reasons why this may happen. Commonly, it's because the organ isn't good enough to be transplanted. The inferior quality of the organ may be discovered during organ procurement or after the organ arrives at the transplant hospital.

wearing a hospital gown most of the time. You'll also be moving between different locations within the hospital — from the preoperative unit to the operating room to the ICU to the nursing floor. If you need something after surgery, your caregiver will be able to bring it to you.

It may be helpful to have a second bag packed in case of a dry run. For this bag, pack medical items and other things you use daily, such as your blood pressure monitor or blood sugar testing equipment. Also bring enough of your prescription medicines and medical supplies for a day or two in case you need to stay overnight somewhere before going back home.

Your caregiver should pack a bag too. The wait may be several hours waiting while you are in surgery. Your caregiver doesn't have to stay in the hospital. They can wait at your hotel or temporary residence as long as they can come to the hospital quickly once your surgery is over. However, if staying at the hospital, your caregiver should pack essentials such as personal medicines, device chargers, warm layers, and reading materials or something to occupy their time while waiting.

During surgery to remove the organ from the donor, the surgeon may see that there's something physically wrong with the organ, a concept dubbed "the eyeball test." Some organs, seemingly healthy, may have scars or lumps in them, which could be a problem. Livers may have fat deposits or signs of cirrhosis, or they may be too big for the recipient. Kidneys and pancreases may have hardened arteries that connect them to the body. Hearts may have problems with blood vessels, and lungs may have damage or infections. Some organs may be damaged by the wear and tear of age but still can be transplanted.

Your transplant team will carefully weigh the benefits and risks of the donated organ. They may decide to move ahead with the transplant because the issues are minor and manageable, or they may deem the risks too great to proceed with the surgery.

Getting the long-awaited call and rushing to the hospital only to go home without the new organ can be emotionally challenging. You may feel that you're back to where you started or that you'll never get a transplant.

These feelings can take a toll on your mental health. This is when transplant support groups can be helpful. Someone in your group may have had a similar experience — and ultimately ended up with a better offer. Listening to their stories may give you a new perspective and help boost your spirits. Transplantation is a complex surgery that involves a difficult recovery. It's important that the organ you receive is healthy and compatible with your system.

Dry runs also can be a learning experience. You've tested your own readiness. You've packed your bags and made arrangements for things to happen in your absence. You've made your trip to the hospital, testing your route and transportation method, and how long it takes to arrive. You know where to go and what to expect when you get your next call.

FOR CAREGIVERS: IT'S GO TIME

Receiving the transplant call can be both thrilling and nerve-racking. On the one hand, it's the moment you and the person in your care have been waiting for. On the other hand, it's time to put your plans for this moment in motion.

There's much work to do. You may need to inform your employer that you're taking time off from work, you may need to contact child care providers and people who watch after your pet or house, and you need to prepare for travel.

You also may need to help your loved one, who may be excited, anxious or apprehensive. Your loved one may feel overwhelmed and have trouble focusing on getting ready. You can help by double-checking the packing list and making sure your loved one has everything needed for the surgery and recovery (see pages 141-142).

You also may need to organize last-minute travel arrangements. If you're driving to the transplant center, make sure the car is gassed up and your bags are in the trunk. Before you leave, run the typical departure checks — the stove is off, doors are locked, and so on.

If you're flying to the transplant center, purchase your airline tickets — or change your departure date and time if you've already purchased flexible tickets — as soon as your transplant team tells you to come to the hospital. You can do this online or by calling the airline. If you're shopping for tickets while your loved one is on standby, some airlines will hold your reservation for 24 hours, and others may allow you to cancel your paid reservation for a full refund within a certain period. Make sure to book a car at your destination or have an alternative transportation method to the hospital.

Your own bags also should be nearly packed and ready to go. Keep in mind that hospitals tend to be cold, so you may want to bring a sweater or a light jacket with you. Consider dressing in layers for going in and out of the hospital. Be sure to pack your own medicines, in addition to your loved one's medicines. If you'll be away from home for a while, make sure you have the items needed for a longer stay.

PACKING CHECKLISTS

Here's what to pack so that you're ready when the time comes. Not all items listed may apply to you.

Transplant recipient's hospital bag

☐ Current medications, including those you may no longer need after transplant.
☐ Eyeglasses or contact lenses and solution.
☐ Hearing aids.
☐ Dentures and related supplies.
☐ Toothbrush and toothpaste.
☐ Personal toiletries.
☐ Cellphone and other digital devices you'll be using.
☐ Wall chargers for all devices.
☐ Comfortable clothing.

- ☐ Button-down shirt if you have a chest port.
- ☐ Underwear and socks.
- ☐ Slip-on shoes with grip (no flip-flops).
- ☐ Wallet or purse.
- ☐ Insurance card.

Transplant recipient's extended-stay packing list

If you'll be recovering away from home, you'll need some extra items. They may include:

Medical items
- ☐ Medical supplies such as oxygen, catheters, ostomy bags, dialysis supplies, wound care supplies and any other items you use daily.
- ☐ Diabetes supplies such as glucometer, pen or testing supplies.
- ☐ Continuous positive airway pressure machine (CPAP) if you use one.
- ☐ Blood pressure cuff.
- ☐ Thermometer, oral or digital.
- ☐ Weight scale.
- ☐ Pill boxes if you use them.
- ☐ Walking aids, such as a walker or a cane, if you use them.

Clothing
- ☐ Additional pairs of comfortable, loose-fitting pants and T-shirts.
- ☐ Additional button-down shirts if you have a chest port.
- ☐ Pajamas, underwear and socks.
- ☐ Weather-appropriate outerwear.
- ☐ Slippers.

Personal items
- ☐ Additional toiletries.
- ☐ Washcloths and towels.
- ☐ Other digital devices.

FOR CAREGIVERS: PACKING CHECKLISTS

Caregivers will also need to be prepared when the time comes. Here's what to pack (not all items listed may apply to you):

Caregiver's bag

☐ Personal medications and medical supplies used daily.

☐ Eyeglasses or contact lenses and solution.

☐ Personal toiletries.

☐ Purse or wallet.

☐ Personal identification document.

☐ Cellphone and other digital devices you'll be using.

☐ Wall chargers for all devices.

☐ Headphones.

☐ Extension cord.

☐ Books, crossword puzzles, knitting or other sources of entertainment.

☐ Favorite snacks.

☐ Water bottle or thermos or both.

☐ Comfortable clothing, including warm layers for cooler environments.

☐ Comfortable shoes and socks.

Caregiver's extended-stay bag

Caregivers who will be away from home for an extended period may want to pack these extra items:

☐ Driver's license if you'll be driving.

☐ Proof of car insurance if you'll be driving.

☐ Your medical insurance card in case you need to see a doctor.

☐ Additional comfortable clothes.

☐ Pajamas, socks and underwear.

☐ Slippers.

☐ Weather-appropriate outerwear.

☐ Additional toiletries.

☐ Washcloths and towels.

☐ Other digital devices.

☐ Any other personal items used daily.

10

In the operating room

You've gotten the call, accepted the offer and the donor organ has been evaluated and determined to be healthy.

When a donor organ is deemed usable for a transplant recipient, the next step is transplant surgery. What happens in the operating room and how long the procedure lasts depend on the organ or organs being transplanted. But first, there's a general preparation that everyone goes through.

PREPPING FOR SURGERY

After you've gone through the hospital admission and registration, a nurse prepares you for your surgery. This includes changing into a hospital gown and removing anything you're wearing, such as glasses, contact lenses, dentures and jewelry.

Afterward, a nurse will use a fine needle to insert a thin plastic tube into a vein in your hand or arm — a procedure often referred to as starting an IV. Medical staff administer medicines and fluids through this tube during the operation.

You'll also meet with some members of your surgical team. They'll explain what they're going to do during surgery and answer your questions. Your anesthesiologist, the person responsible for keeping you asleep during surgery, will explain other IVs or catheters you may need. Your surgical team also will ask you to sign consent papers stating you're aware of the risks and benefits of the surgery and that you agree to have the surgery.

You may feel anxious or apprehensive during this preparation. You also may feel relieved that your wait's finally over and you're about to cross this major milestone you've been preparing for. Your caregiver and other family members can stay with you during your prep time, so they can help you with instructions and any potentially challenging moments.

While you're being prepped for surgery, your surgical team will be getting ready too. They'll be reviewing the operation and scrubbing in — sterilizing their hands and putting on sterile gowns and gloves to reduce the risk of infection.

A transplant surgical team generally consists of several people:
- The transplant surgeon and a surgical assistant or surgical trainee.
- An anesthesiologist and a nurse anesthetist or an anesthesiology trainee.
- A surgical technician responsible for handling instruments during surgery.
- Circulating nurses who may go in and out of the operating room to bring various items if needed, such as medicines, blood transfusion packs or additional instruments.
- Medical students or other healthcare professionals in training.

When you're brought to the operating room, you'll be placed on the operating table. After a few minutes, you'll be given medicine that lets you sleep through the surgery. Once you're asleep, your team will further prepare you for the procedure. They'll connect soft, thin IV tubes to blood vessels in your neck and arms to give you medicine and fluids. Other tubes will be used to monitor your body's vital signs. A tube called a catheter will be placed in your bladder to drain urine until you're able to use the toilet again.

The anesthesiologist will place a soft plastic tube down your throat so that a ventilator can pump air to your lungs during the surgery. Depending on the type of transplant you're receiving, you may need additional tubes and monitoring devices.

Your surgical team also will give you some medicines through your IV connection, including antibiotics to prevent infections and your first dose of antirejection medication. This first dose, sometimes referred to as induction, contains powerful antirejection medicines to prevent your immune system from going into overdrive and rejecting the organ after it's been grafted to your body.

Lastly, your team will do a final check, sometimes called a time-out, to verify everything is ready. They'll also run through a surgical checklist of what needs to be done. After that, your surgery will begin.

Depending on the type of transplant you're receiving, your surgeon will make different incisions in different parts of your body and will perform various tasks. All transplanted organs need a reliable blood supply, so your surgeon will connect the organ to your arteries and veins, as well as to other parts of your body. Because some organs take longer to connect than others, time spent in the operating room varies from patient to patient.

KIDNEY TRANSPLANT SURGERY

If you're receiving a kidney from a living donor, your surgery and your donor's surgery will take place at about the same time. But you won't be in the same operating room. If you're receiving a kidney from a deceased donor, your organ may already have arrived in the operating room. A kidney transplant surgery usually takes 2 to 4 hours.

It may sound surprising, but in most cases, a surgeon will leave your own kidneys in place. Your kidneys are removed only if they're inflamed, swollen, causing pain or diseased — as in the case of poly-cystic kidney disease, for example. But if your kidneys simply aren't working well, they'll be left where they are. Removing them would create a bigger, and often unnecessary, surgery. Your surgeon will try to avoid that if possible. Instead, your new kidney will be placed in your lower abdomen.

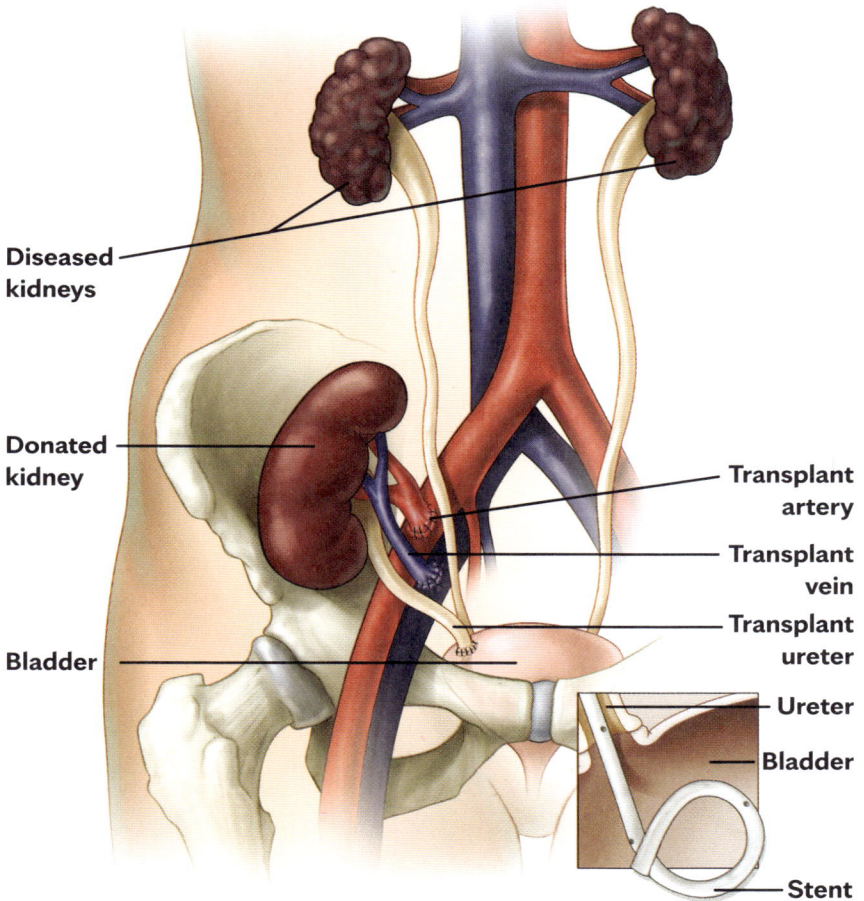

Most often, the diseased kidneys are left in place, and the new kidney is placed nearby. The new kidney's artery and vein are connected to the recipient's main leg artery and vein. The new kidney's ureter, which carries urine from the kidney, is connected to the recipient's bladder, often with a stent in place to promote proper healing.

To transplant the new kidney, an incision is made in your lower abdomen. The surgeon locates the blood vessels leading to your legs. Your new kidney needs to be connected to these blood vessels so it can filter toxins and waste products from your blood. Your surgeon will temporarily clamp your vessels to stop the blood flow and then connect these vessels to the transplanted kidney's blood vessels.

Once blood vessels are stitched together, the clamps are removed so that blood can flow to your new kidney. The transplanted kidney should turn rosy or "pink up," a sign that blood is flowing appropriately. The kidney may start making urine shortly after, or it may take a few days to "wake up" and begin working.

Your surgeon also must connect your new kidney to your bladder. A tube called a ureter channels urine from the kidney to the bladder. The transplanted kidney's ureter is connected to your bladder with stitches. A small piece of soft plastic tubing called a stent may be placed inside the ureter to help the connection heal. The stent usually stays there for several weeks and is removed later through a noninvasive procedure.

LIVER TRANSPLANT SURGERY

If you're receiving part of a liver from a living donor, the two surgeries will be performed at about the same time, but you won't be in the same operating room. If you're receiving a liver from a deceased donor, it may already be in the operating room or it may arrive there shortly after your surgery begins. Liver transplant surgery is complex and can take 4 to 12 hours.

To begin the procedure, a long incision is made in the upper half of your abdomen. The location and size of the incision depends on your surgeon's approach and your anatomy. For liver transplant, the diseased liver must be removed before the new liver is transplanted. The surgery is performed the same way regardless of whether the new liver is from a deceased donor or a living donor. The entire diseased liver is removed, and the donor liver is placed in the same location where the diseased liver was.

Removing the liver can be a difficult procedure because it's a large organ with many blood vessels attached to it, so it can bleed easily. Some people undergoing a liver transplant will need a blood

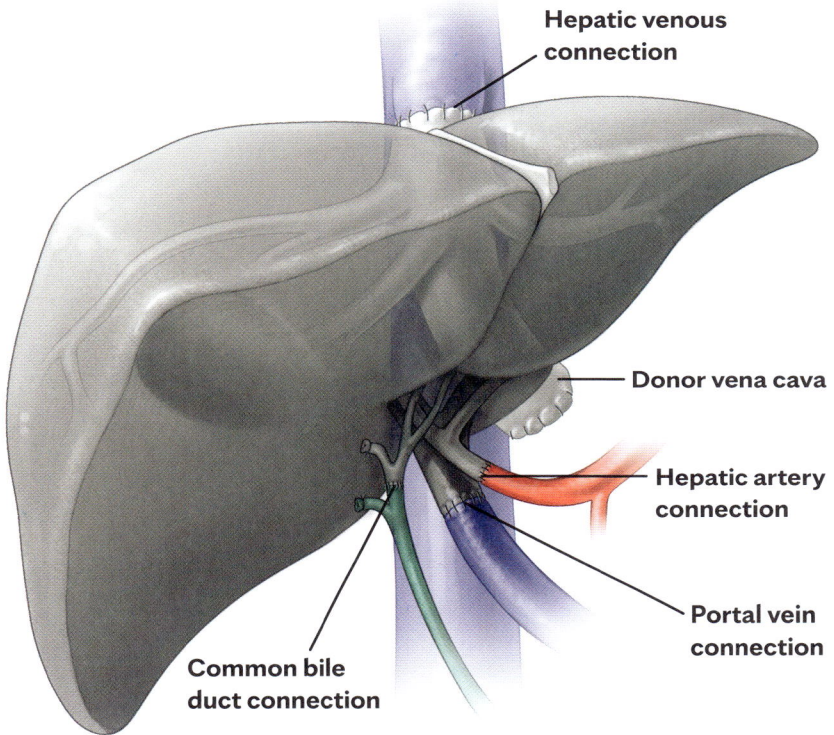

Hepatic venous connection

Donor vena cava

Hepatic artery connection

Portal vein connection

Common bile duct connection

Donor anatomy represented in gray

To work properly, the new liver must be connected to your body's blood vessels and bile ducts or small intestine.

transfusion. Sometimes your own blood spilling into the abdomen may be collected during surgery and recirculated back into your bloodstream.

Your new liver is attached to your body's blood vessels. It also needs to be connected to your bile ducts so that bile — the digestive liquid the liver makes — can flow into your bowel. If your bile ducts

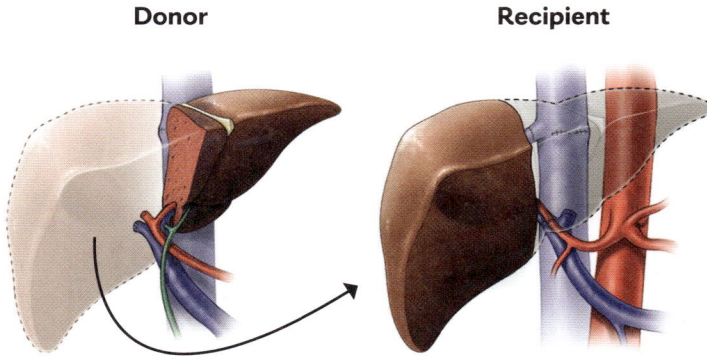

Donor   Recipient

Approximately 60% of the donor's liver is used for transplant in a living-donor liver donation.

are too small or are damaged, the surgeon will connect the donor liver ducts directly to your intestine.

Because bile ducts take some time to heal, a temporary draining tube may be put in place that's typically removed within a month after surgery. Other tubes may be placed in your abdomen to drain fluids during and after surgery. These will be removed gradually as you recover.

The medical team will monitor your oxygen level, blood pressure and the pressure inside your heart's chambers. The team also will run several blood tests during the surgery to see how well your blood is clotting. Sometimes, they may give you additional blood products, such as plasma or platelets, to help with clotting.

HEART TRANSPLANT SURGERY

Heart transplant surgery is performed through an incision in the front of your chest and can take 5 to 8 hours. If you've had previous heart surgeries, opening your chest may take longer as the team carefully works around previous scars and any scar tissue. If you're using a ventricular assist device, which is a pump that's implanted to keep your heart beating, it will likely take extra time to remove the device.

Accessing your heart requires cutting through your chest bone. Your surgeon first will open your chest with an incision down the midline of your breastbone and then will cut through that breastbone using a specialized device. This procedure is called a sternotomy. It allows the surgeon to access your heart and perform the transplant procedure. Your diseased heart must be removed before transplanting a new heart.

To maintain blood supply to the rest of your organs, the team will use a heart-lung machine. Your main arteries are connected to the machine, which takes over the function of the heart and lungs to deliver oxygen to your body during the operation.

A catheter will be placed into your heart through blood vessels in your neck to monitor your heart function after surgery. The catheter is

HEART TRANSPLANT

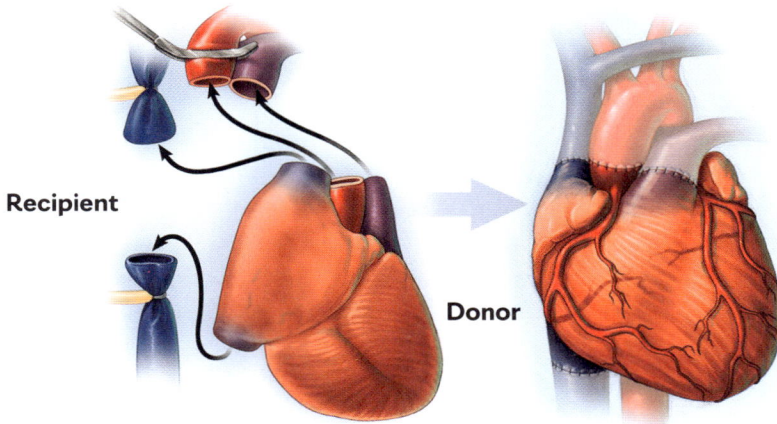

Recipient

Donor

The donor heart is attached to the recipient's blood vessels. Once blood flows in, the donor heart often starts pumping right away.

removed once your team is satisfied that your new heart is working as it should.

Once your new heart is attached to your blood vessels and blood flow is restored, the new heart often starts beating on its own. If it doesn't start beating right away, your surgeon may give it a slight electrical shock, similar to a shock from a defibrillator. Once your surgeon is satisfied with how your new heart is pumping, the heart-lung machine is disconnected, and the incision is closed.

LUNG TRANSPLANT SURGERY

Where incisions are made and how many incisions are needed for a lung transplant depends on your specific anatomy and whether you're getting a single- or double-lung transplant. These factors also determine the duration of the surgery. For a single-lung transplant, your surgery may take 6 to 8 hours. A double-lung transplant may take 8 to 12 hours.

With a single-lung transplant, an incision generally is made on the side of your chest with the diseased lung. This incision may be under the breast fold and toward the back. Sometimes a single-lung transplant requires a sternotomy, in which the breastbone is cut in two, similar to heart transplant surgery.

For a double-lung transplant, a horizontal incision typically is made across the entire chest, from one underarm to the other. The surgeon will then split the breastbone and enter the chest cavity between the ribs to remove the diseased lungs and replace them with new lungs. Other techniques that are better suited to a person's anatomy sometimes may be used.

Similar to a heart transplant, you may need the help of a machine to circulate your blood and oxygen. Your team will put you either on a heart-lung machine or another device called ECMO, which stands for extracorporeal membrane oxygenation. ECMO removes carbon dioxide and sends oxygen-rich blood back to the body, so you don't have to use your own lungs for a period of time.

Removal of a diseased lung requires it to be separated from the heart and chest wall. This is a delicate and complex procedure because the lungs are surrounded by other important organs, including the diaphragm, esophagus and vocal cord nerves. Your surgeon will

Single-lung transplant

Recipient

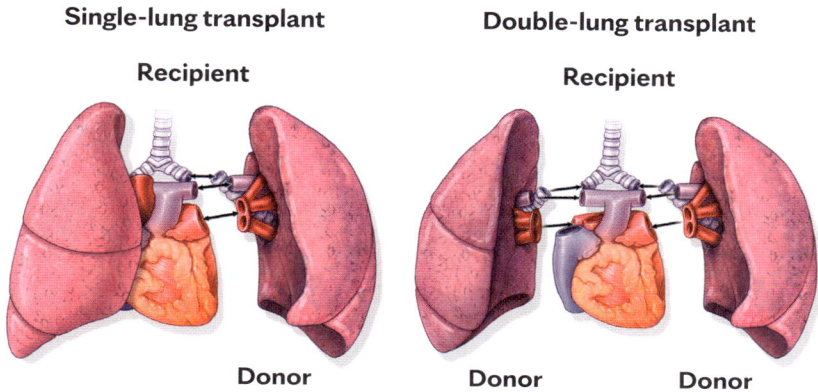

Donor

Double-lung transplant

Recipient

Donor   Donor

A lung transplant may replace one or both lungs.

carefully detach your lung from your heart and airway. Then the surgeon will connect the new donor lung to your airway and the blood vessels leading to the heart. If you're having a double-lung transplant, the same procedure is repeated on the other side.

When the connections are made, blood flow is restored to the lungs to begin to ventilate them. Once the lungs are working as they should, the incisions are closed. However, various drainage tubes will remain in your chest and be removed later as you recover.

PANCREAS TRANSPLANT SURGERY

Pancreas transplant surgery usually lasts about 3 to 6 hours, depending on whether you're having a pancreas transplant alone or receiving a new pancreas and a new kidney at the same time.

Similar to a kidney transplant, a pancreas transplant doesn't require your pancreas to be removed. Your new pancreas will be placed inside your abdominal cavity. The surgeon will make a long incision in your abdomen and find your blood vessels. The blood vessels of the donor pancreas are connected with your blood vessels so that the new pancreas can secrete insulin into your bloodstream.

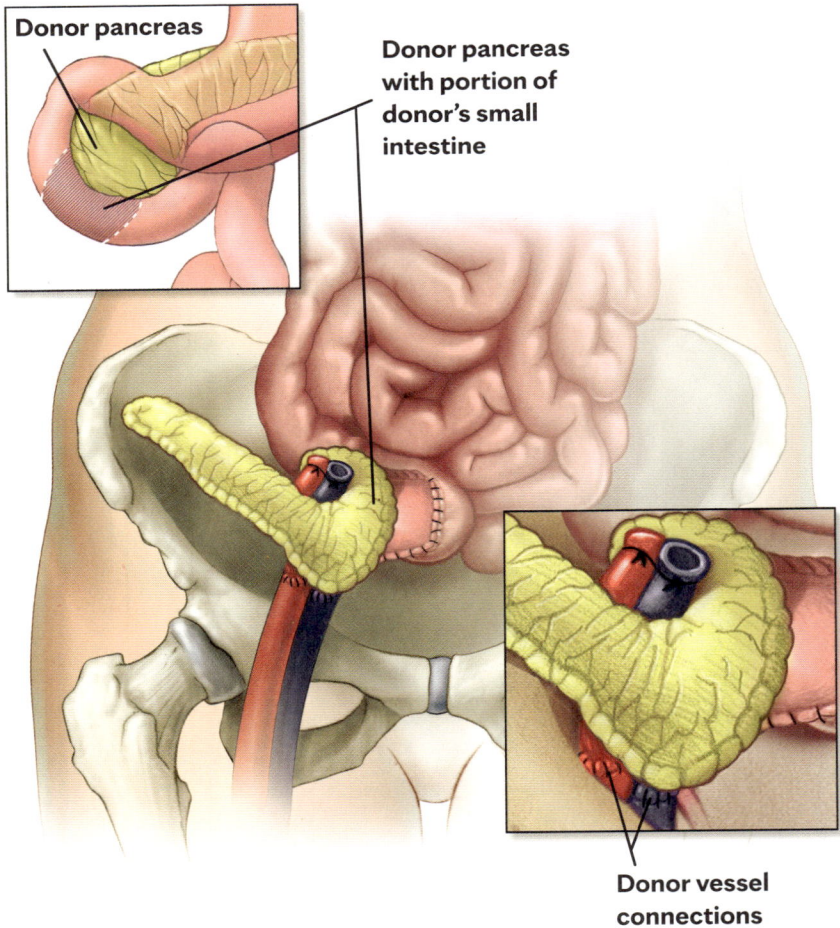

Donor pancreas

Donor pancreas with portion of donor's small intestine

Donor vessel connections

During transplant surgery, the donor pancreas and a small portion of the donor's small intestine are placed into the recipient's lower abdomen. The donor intestine is attached to either the small intestine or the bladder and the donor pancreas is connected to blood vessels that also supply blood to the legs.

In addition to making insulin, the pancreas makes digestive chemicals called enzymes, which flow into the intestines. The donor pancreas will have a piece of the donor intestine attached to it. Your surgeon will connect the piece of donor intestine to your intestine so chemicals from the donor pancreas drain directly into your intestines.

As blood flows into the new pancreas, it should "pink up" and start producing insulin. Your blood sugar should start to regulate very quickly. When the new organ appears to be working as expected, the incision in your abdomen is closed.

FOR CAREGIVERS: WHILE YOU WAIT

Your loved one has just left for the operating room. Now what?

Of all the parts of the transplant journey, this is the only one where you'll have nothing to do but wait. Yet waiting can be excruciating, especially if your loved one is undergoing a longer surgery, such as a liver or double-lung transplant. If your loved one's surgery is only a few hours, you can wait at the hospital. But if it's a longer transplant, you may want to go back home or to the hotel where you're staying. Whichever you choose, make sure the healthcare team knows how to contact you.

If you choose to wait in the hospital, bring something to keep yourself occupied, such as a book. Bring an extra layer of clothing with you, as hospital air can be cold. To pass time, go for a walk, buy yourself some food, or chat with friends and family.

If you choose to wait at the location where you're staying, try taking a nap or a bath. If you have access to a kitchen, you may want to make meals for yourself for the upcoming days because you'll spend most of your time in the hospital with your loved one. And if you're feeling anxious or apprehensive, try listening to calming music, meditating, exercising or any activity that helps you relax.

11

Recovery after surgery

A MISS, COMPLICATIONS AND A FULL RECOVERY
KRISTINE'S STORY

As a young woman, Kristine experienced several autoimmune conditions and learned to deal with pain and discomfort. Things got worse in her mid-30s when she developed primary biliary cirrhosis, a chronic autoimmune liver disease that damages the bile ducts. "I was diagnosed in 2008," she says. "I didn't start getting sick until 2016," she adds. But she was told that there may come a time when she would need a transplant.

That time came three years later in 2019, when Kristine started feeling progressively worse. Primary biliary cirrhosis caused ascites, which is fluid accumulation inside the stomach. Kristine was losing weight, feeling nauseous and had to have fluids drained from inside her belly multiple times a week. It was clear that she needed a new liver. Eventually, Kristine was listed for a transplant in her state.

She waited for the transplant call, but things moved slowly, and she was growing sicker. Kristine and her husband decided to look elsewhere. "We had a friend who was transplanted at Mayo Clinic, and I found out they took my insurance," she says.

After her evaluation, Kristine returned home to get ready to temporarily relocate. She wanted to be near the hospital when she received the call. "I came back home to see my kids because I knew I wasn't going to see them for their birthdays," she says. "I came home and had a birthday party for them, not really thinking I would get a call so quickly." Unfortunately, she wasn't able to make it back in time. "I missed the call, which was really hard," she shares. "So, we went down the next day, and within two weeks, I had another call, and I had my transplant."

Kristine, however, encountered some hurdles in her transplant journey, eventually requiring additional surgeries. During her recoveries, Kristine had to rely on different caregivers at different times, including her mother, her husband, a friend, and even her two daughters. Adjusting to post-transplant life was challenging, particularly learning to manage the medicines. "It took me a little while to learn. It was weeks before I really started to do them on my own," she says. "My mom did all my medication management at first. But once I started doing them myself, it was really easy."

The hardest part of the transplant journey wasn't the pain or the uncertainty of her situation, but the fact that Kristine couldn't see her family. "I wasn't used to being away from my kids and my grandson," she says. "Thank goodness for FaceTime so I could talk to my husband and my kids."

Introducing the necessary dietary and social safety elements into her post-transplant life took some work too. Her family adopted a Mediterranean diet to stay healthy. "There's no binge eating," she shares. There's no just grabbing a sandwich at a deli because the food may be contaminated with bacteria after sitting in the open for a while. "At work, we have a lot of potlucks," she adds, which she can't partake in either. "I don't know who brought the food, who touched it, so I can't have it."

Transplant support groups were tremendously helpful, Kristine notes. "They were a saving grace," she says, adding that the group still stays in touch. "Now we do it on Zoom, and there are people all over the United States who have lots of different stories. We all are grateful to Jenna, the social worker who created such a gentle and calm community so we all can talk."

Kristine wholeheartedly recommends transplant support groups to everyone on a transplant journey. "I would definitely tell people to attend the support groups, because it's a great place to learn about all the things that can happen prior to transplant, after transplant and during transplant."

Another piece of advice from Kristine is to follow the transplant care team's directions exactly. "Listen to the doctors. They know what they're talking about. Do what they're telling you, and you'll get there," she says. "I just had blood work yesterday. My numbers all look incredible. I'm doing well and I'm here for my children and grandchildren."

When you wake up after your surgery, you likely won't remember much. You may remember being prepped for surgery or the last few moments before falling asleep, or you may not remember either. The medicines used for anesthesia can interfere with your memory in some ways. They also can make you feel groggy, sleepy and disoriented. All of that is expected.

WAKING UP
If you've received a kidney or pancreas transplant, you'll likely wake up in a postoperative recovery unit. If your surgery was uncomplicated, you won't remain connected to a ventilator or have a breathing tube in your throat. A recovery nurse will be waiting for you to awaken, and you should be able to speak right away.

For other transplants you'll likely wake up in the intensive care unit (ICU). If you don't awaken on your own and your vitals show that you're doing well, your transplant team will gently try to wake you after several hours.

You still may be intubated when you first awaken. Most people, however, don't have any awareness of this part of their recovery. Being intubated means that you're connected to a ventilator machine that's pumping air into your lungs through a breathing tube inserted into your throat. You won't be able to talk, eat or drink right away, so you'll receive fluids and nourishment through an IV. You'll also have a catheter

YOUR POST-TRANSPLANT CARE TEAM

The following individuals will likely be involved in your care while you're in the hospital and during your recovery afterward.

- **Transplant surgeon and transplant nephrologist (kidney, pancreas), hepatologist (liver), cardiologist (heart) or pulmonologist (lungs).** The care team regularly reviews your test results and adjusts your medicines as needed.
- **Bedside nurse.** This person helps you with wound care, blood tests, pain, medicines, insulin injections, if needed, and other care. Nursing staff also educate you about things that you'll need to do once you leave the hospital, including measuring your blood pressure and blood sugar.
- **Inpatient nurse coordinator.** A nurse coordinator makes sure that you receive your medicines from the pharmacy and have information about each medicine you need to take. This person also makes sure you have a schedule of your follow-up appointments.
- **Inpatient transplant social worker.** A social worker can assist you with unexpected issues and challenges after surgery, including managing stress and other emotions.
- **Physical therapist and occupational therapist.** These individuals can help you regain your strength and mobility, as well as your breathing capacity.
- **Case manager.** A case manager is responsible for discharge planning and home healthcare.

draining urine from your bladder. Your hands may be held down with soft restraints. This is done so that you don't accidentally pull the breathing tube out or pull out any other tubes that you're connected to. This can be frustrating, but it's a necessary precaution to keep you safe during your recovery. It's likely that you won't be aware of this part of your recovery because of the medicines you'll be receiving.

If all your vital signs remain stable once you're awake, you'll be taken off the ventilator, and the breathing tube will be removed. The length of time that you're on a ventilator depends on the organ being transplanted. On average, people receiving a heart are on a ventilator 1 to 2 days after the surgery. Lung recipients may be on a ventilator for several days. Your throat may feel a little sore, and you may sound hoarse once the breathing tube is removed. But these side effects tend to go away quickly.

There may be other tubes connected to your body, including those that drain fluid from the surgical site. And you may be attached to wires as well. For example, in the case of a heart transplant, you'll have wires attached to your heart that exit out of your chest. On the outside, the wires are attached to an external pacemaker. A transplanted heart may beat slower than usual for the first few days, so the pacemaker helps it keep pace. For most heart recipients, these wires are removed within a couple of weeks.

Don't be surprised if you feel bloated after your operation, and your bowels may not work right away. These things are common after surgery. This is partially due to the effects of anesthesia. Also, with certain types of transplants, the surgeon must rearrange your bowels during surgery.

Your transplant care team will likely prescribe medicines to help get your bowels moving again, but these take time to work. Your care team will encourage you to be up in a chair and even walking as early as possible after surgery. This helps improve the function of the intestines and also helps keep your lungs healthy and reduces the risk of blood clots forming in the veins of your legs.

It's also common to experience pain after transplant surgery. You'll be given medicines to lessen the pain and help you sleep.

If you're doing well after the first few days, you'll be transferred from the ICU to a regular care unit. Leaving the ICU means that your health is improving. Congratulations — you now have a working organ and things are looking up!

GETTING BACK ON YOUR FEET

Not long after surgery, your care team will work to get you moving again, even though you may still feel sleepy, groggy or sluggish. If you've received a donor kidney or liver, typically you'll sit in a chair or stand up and maybe even take your first steps around the room within a day — and then down the hospital hallway. The goal will be to take several such walks daily.

This may sound like a rapid transition, but research finds that the longer people remain inactive after surgery, the longer it takes for them to recover. On the other hand, the sooner you start moving, the faster you're likely to bounce back. Moving sooner rather than later also decreases the chances of developing blood clots, which could lead to serious complications. So even though you may feel dizzy or sore, focus on doing what you can to start moving. This will boost your chances of going home in a timely manner.

Your care team also will help you manage your pain level. The lingering effects of anesthesia can protect you from postsurgical pain for a short time, such as a day or two. Once that protective effect wears off, you may feel worse than you did when you first woke up — and it may feel like a setback. Often, the third and fourth days after surgery can feel like the worst days in terms of pain. Once you get through them, you should start feeling better.

While some level of discomfort is expected during your recovery, you shouldn't be in pain, and pain shouldn't keep you from moving about. It's important to minimize your pain because that helps you recover faster. If you feel that your pain is becoming too much to handle, let your transplant team know.

As you begin moving, a physical therapist will work with you to regain some of the abilities you had before surgery. For example, heart and lung transplant recipients undergo specific breathing, coughing and cardiovascular exercises. An occupational therapist can help restore your hand and grip strength. Heart or lung surgery can affect movements of muscles in the hand.

As for your diet, you should be able to start eating regular foods once you're off the ventilator or shortly after surgery if you're not on a ventilator. If you're having trouble swallowing, you may have to begin with softer foods, such as applesauce. Depending on your transplant type and your specific situation, your diet may need to be adjusted. For example, you may initially be on a low-salt diet to help decrease fluid buildup. Your transplant care team will work with you to set your dietary arrangements.

A RECOVERY PLAN

Your care team may put together a recovery plan for the first few days after surgery. This type of plan generally outlines activities that you might expect to do on Day 1, Day 2, and so on. Some of these activities you may be able to do by yourself. Other activities may require the help of your caregiver, a nurse or your care team.

A recovery plan the first couple of days after surgery may look something like this, depending on the organ you have transplanted. A person receiving a donor kidney may leave the hospital in two or three days, whereas a person receiving a donor heart will be in the hospital longer.

Day 1
- Bathe, brush your teeth and comb your hair, with help from your caregiver or a member of the care team if needed.
- Walk or sit in a chair at least 3 to 4 times during the day, with assistance. You must be able to walk safely before you can leave the hospital.
- Determine the foods you can eat and order meals from a menu.

MEDICINES AND MONITORING

Medicines are key to your recovery and to your overall transplant success. After surgery you'll likely receive medicine through an IV. Once the transplant team feels comfortable with the recovery of your bowel function, you'll switch to medicines taken by mouth. Your medicines and their dosages will be adjusted by your care team depending on your progress and the results of your blood work. It's important to keep track of these changes so that when you leave the hospital you're taking the right medicines in the right amounts. You'll be taking many different medicines, which may include:

- Start learning about the medicines prescribed for you and how to take them.

Day 2
- Get instructions on how to care for your incision while in the shower. Your transplant team will help you if necessary.
- Walk at least six times during the day, with assistance if necessary.
- Meet with a rehabilitation specialist to discuss exercises that are important for you to do as part of your recovery.
- Get instructions on how to manage a catheter or drain if you'll be leaving the hospital with a catheter or drain.

As your strength improves, your transplant team will work with you to further develop your recovery plan until you're ready to be discharged from the hospital.

Your recovery plan also may include tasks for your caregiver, including starting a record book that includes your lab results, your vital signs and a schedule of the medicines you need to take, including the doses.

- **Antirejection medicines.** Also known as immunosuppressants, these medicines prevent rejection of your new organ.
- **Steroids.** They may be part of your antirejection regimen. You may need to take steroids for a time, but the goal is to minimize steroid use because of the side effects. Some medical centers offer steroid-free regimens.
- **Antibiotics and antiviral medicines.** They're taken to prevent the development of an infection.
- **Pain medicines.** They help keep you comfortable and allow you to move about.

MEDICINES TO PREVENT REJECTION

Antirejection medicines are generally taken twice a day, 12 hours apart. Some of the more commonly used medicines include the following:

- Tacrolimus (Prograf, Astagraf XL, Envarsus XR).
- Sirolimus (Rapamune).
- Cyclosporine (Sandimmune, Neoral, Gengraf).
- Mycophenolate mofetil (CellCept, Myhibbin).
- Everolimus (Afinitor, Zortress).
- Prednisone.

Which of these medicines you take depends on several factors, including how well your body tolerates the medicine, how well it works and its side effects. Your transplant team will put together a regimen that works best for you. By the time you go home, you'll have your medicine routine in place. As you recover, adjustments likely will be made to match your needs.

Make sure to order refills of these medicines at least 1 to 2 weeks in advance so that you don't run out. Antirejection medicines are crucial to a successful transplant.

The medicines can be expensive. If your insurance coverage changes, you can no longer afford your medicines, or you're about to run out without any refills, notify your transplant care team as soon as possible. Your care team can assist in finding resources for you. You need to take these medicines every day.

Managing side effects

Unfortunately, many of the medicines you take can have side effects. Steroids and tacrolimus, for example, can both cause high blood pressure and high blood sugar, so you may need additional medicines to regulate your blood pressure, blood sugar or both, as well as temporary insulin injections.

Steroids also can cause insomnia, jitteriness, shakiness, confusion and mood swings. These symptoms tend to improve as the dosage is reduced, and some may be helped by sleep medicines or antidepressants. You also may benefit from calcium and magnesium supplements because steroids can affect the balance of these compounds in your body.

Some medicines can cause kidney damage, so your transplant care team will check your kidney function regularly and adjust your medicines as necessary. You can read more about medicines in Chapter 13.

Monitoring your new organ
After surgery, X-rays, ultrasound or other images will be taken of your transplanted organ to make sure it's functioning and healthy.

A biopsy may be taken of your new organ as part of the routine assessment of the organ. A biopsy also may be done if there is a concern about the organ's functioning or the potential for rejection. A biopsy is a procedure to remove a small sample of tissue for testing in a laboratory. This is done to determine whether the newly grafted tissue is being accepted by your body or if there's a risk of rejection.

For most organs, a thin needle is used to take a few tissue samples of your new kidney, liver or pancreas. For a heart biopsy, a thin plastic tube equipped with a tiny tweezers is threaded through a small incision in one of your blood vessels to the heart. For a lung biopsy, the tissue sample is generally obtained during a procedure called bronchoscopy.

In the past, biopsies were done about once a week during the recovery period. Today, new and improved blood tests often replace biopsies, making the rejection monitoring process easier and less invasive. If your transplant care team determines that there's a risk of rejection or you're experiencing rejection, they'll adjust your antirejection medicines or give you IV medicines to treat the rejection.

Your transplant care team also will help you understand what your medicines do, what doses you need, and when and how to take them. As you recover, this information may change, sometimes daily. Be sure to follow the instructions from your care team, as the information printed on your medicine bottles may become outdated. Consider keeping track of your current medication regimen in a notebook,

UNDERSTANDING REJECTION AND HOW IT'S MANAGED

After transplant, there's always a risk of rejection of the new organ. Fortunately, modern medicine is very good at minimizing this risk. There are three types of rejection:

Hyperacute transplant rejection

Hyperacute transplant rejection occurs within minutes or hours after the transplant. It happens when preformed antibodies against the donor organ are present in high amounts. That reaction is similar to what happens when a person is given a blood transfusion of the wrong blood type. Luckily this type of rejection almost never happens because transplant recipients with preformed antibodies undergo a series of tests to find well-matched donors.

Acute transplant rejection

Acute transplant rejection results when your body's immune system identifies the transplanted organ as a foreign entity. It can happen even with well-matched donors and recipients. Avoiding an acute transplant rejection is why transplant recipients must take antirejection medications for the rest of their lives. Modern antirejection medicines are very effective. As long as you take them every day, your chances of avoiding rejection are very good.

Chronic transplant rejection

Chronic transplant rejection may develop over time, particularly when transplant recipients don't have regular lab tests or if they miss taking doses of their antirejection medication. Without regular monitoring, a person's antibody levels may increase higher than what's considered optimal. They may have been experiencing a level of rejection for some time. Untreated, this can lead to gradual wear and tear on the organ. Adjusting your antirejection medicines can prevent chronic transplant rejection. This is why attending all follow-up appointments is so important.

where you write down the dates, medicine names, doses and changes as you go.

You also can use your notebook to keep track of questions you may have, such as about the progress of your recovery, side effects of your medicines or management of your pain. Nursing staff often can help answer many of these questions. If you have a question for your surgeon, attending physician or other transplant care specialist, it may help to keep in mind that these individuals usually make their rounds in the morning. Having your questions ready at this time can help get your questions answered.

As you recover, you'll be able to gradually reduce or even stop taking some medicines. That means that many side effects you may be experiencing will go away. However, in the early days of living with your new organ, taking all your medicines exactly as prescribed, including following any adjustments made by your team, is crucial.

GETTING DISCHARGED FROM THE HOSPITAL

The length of time it takes to recover from a transplant surgery depends on the type of organ transplant received. For example, it's not uncommon to go home with a new kidney just a few days after surgery. Hospital stays after other types of transplants may be longer. For example, you're likely to stay in the hospital a week for a liver or pancreas transplant, up to two weeks for a new heart, and up to three weeks for new lungs.

For some people, recovery may take longer still. That doesn't mean your new organ isn't doing well. More likely, it means that your body is recovering at its own pace. Try focusing on your daily exercises, getting stronger, taking your medicines on time and staying positive. Your discharge moment will get closer with each passing day.

To be discharged from the hospital, you must be able to:

- Eat regular food.
- Be strong enough to get out of bed and walk safely.
- Manage your pain.
- Know your medicines and how and when to take them.
- Tolerate your medicines.

YOUR OUTPATIENT APPOINTMENTS

Once you're discharged from the hospital, you'll have many follow-up appointments. You'll see the transplant team regularly for laboratory work, imaging procedures, consultations with the healthcare team, medication adjustments and possibly a biopsy. Here's what to remember.

- With the help of your caregiver, keep track of your scheduled appointments.
- If you have questions, have your caregiver write them down and make notes of the answers for later reference.
- Follow the instructions regarding whether you're allowed to eat before lab tests. Drinking water is OK.
- Don't take your antirejection medications before lab tests. Bring the medicines with you and take them immediately after your tests are done.

If you live near your transplant center, you'll be able to go home from the hospital. If you moved to be closer to your transplant center, you'll return to your temporary residence. Many transplant centers, including those at Mayo Clinic's three main sites, offer low-cost housing for transplant recipients and their caregivers. One of the advantages of these facilities is that you'll have the company of other people going through similar experiences. This can be a strong source of support.

FOR CAREGIVERS: YOU'VE GOT THIS

Helping your loved one through recovery after surgery is likely to be the most demanding part of your transplant journey. At the same time, it's also the most rewarding part of your experience. This is the time when the person you're supporting will need you the most and you can have the most impact.

After surgery your loved one may not be able to communicate effectively for a while. That's where your help is needed. Keep track of the instructions you receive and take notes about test results. Learn as much as you can about your loved one's medicines, doses and side effects. Keep in mind that medicines and doses may change frequently as the team develops the best regimen for your loved one, so make sure to keep your notes up to date.

At the hospital
You'll likely be expected to be at the hospital with your loved one during the day. It's important to be there in the morning when the transplant team is making rounds. Both you and the person in your care may have questions to ask the team. If your loved one is asleep or tired, it's up to you to ask the questions and write down the answers you receive.

Throughout the day, your loved one will need help getting out of bed, standing up, walking around and doing exercises. You also may help your loved one wash up or take a shower and assist with wound care.

If you want to stay with your loved one overnight, that's usually OK. Some caregivers choose to stay because they want to offer round-the-clock support. Others like to do it because they feel it helps them better understand the caregiving routine and what's going on with their loved one's recovery. But caregivers also need rest. If you're not getting sufficient sleep, consider spending the night where you can get a good night's rest. This will help you be a better caregiver. One of the main reasons it's so important for caregivers to get good rest is that recovery after transplant is a long process. Think of it as a marathon, not a sprint.

Keep in mind that once your loved one goes home with you, your caregiver responsibilities will increase as you provide care around the clock. You'll need to drive to appointments, prepare meals and help with self-care. You also need to encourage your loved one to eat well and exercise.

In addition, you'll be an important source of emotional support through pain, exhaustion, medicine side effects and mood swings. Your loved one may feel irritable or agitated and find it difficult to wait for the healing process to unfold. These sentiments are common and often ease as recovery progresses. Do your best to be patient, optimistic and encouraging. Remind the person in your care how far you've come together. Celebrate daily achievements and recovery milestones.

Avoiding burnout

As you continue to provide care, you may find yourself feeling tired, exhausted or depleted. You may realize that you're becoming increasingly irritable, anxious or unhappy. It's important to recognize that these are signs of caregiver burnout. If you allow your health and well-being to deteriorate, it'll affect your caregiving abilities as well as the recovery of the person in your care.

A little self-care can go a long way. If you're staying with your loved one in the hospital at night, consider sleeping at home or at the location where you're staying temporarily. Spend some time doing things you enjoy. Take a walk, watch a funny TV show, or treat yourself to a

SIGNS OF CAREGIVER STRESS AND BURNOUT

As a caregiver, you may be so focused on the person in your care that you may miss the signs that your own health and well-being are taking a hit. The signs of caregiver stress or burnout include:

- Feeling burdened, worried or anxious all the time.
- Feeling tired or exhausted often.
- Feeling sad.
- Sleeping too much or not enough.
- Gaining or losing weight.
- Becoming easily irritated or angry.
- Losing interest in activities you used to enjoy.
- Having frequent headaches or other pains or health problems.
- Missing your own medical appointments.
- Misusing alcohol or drugs, including prescription medicines.

massage or a spa visit. Taking care of yourself is key to taking care of others.

If you find yourself close to a breaking point, ask for help. Join a caregiver support group where you can share your challenges and ask others how they dealt with similar situations. Also consider asking other family members for help, such as with shopping, cleaning or making meals. The emotional and physical demands of caregiving can strain even the strongest person, so don't be afraid to ask for or accept help.

Well-being strategies

The emotional and physical demands of caring for a transplant recipient is a full-time job — and often a stressful one. Here are some tips to help you along the way:

- **Ask for and accept help.** Make a list of ways in which others can help you. Then ask people in your support circles to do some tasks, for example, food shopping, cooking or laundry.
- **Focus on what you can do.** At times, you might feel like you're not doing enough. But no one is a perfect caregiver. You're doing the best you can.
- **Set goals you can reach.** Break large tasks into smaller steps that you can do one at a time. Make lists of what's most important. Follow a daily routine.
- **Seek social support.** Stay in touch with the caregiving support groups in the hospital and online. Reach out to family and friends who support you, even if they can't help you on a daily basis. Make a point of talking to them regularly, sharing your emotions and feelings.
- **Find ways to sleep better.** Try intentionally relaxing your muscles, reading a book or taking a calming bath before bed.
- **Take care of your health.** Exercise when you can. Move as much as possible. Eat a healthy diet and drink plenty of water.

12

Pediatric transplant surgery

GETTING HEALTHY TO HAVE A CHANCE
HANNA'S STORY

Each year on the tenth of March, Hanna's family dons green clothing and bracelets, and they eat green-colored cookies and snacks, among other traditions. It would be easy to confuse these festivities with an early St. Patrick's Day celebration, but this green is different. This green is to celebrate 8-year-old Hanna's second chance at life.

"We consider it like another birthday," says Hanna's mom, Melinda. "March 10 is the day when she received her new liver. We call it her 'liver-versary.' And green is the color of liver disease awareness."

When Hanna was an infant, she was diagnosed with biliary atresia, a rare, life-threatening liver condition that caused her bile ducts to become scarred and blocked. A treatment to bypass the malfunctioning bile ducts, called a Kasai procedure, didn't work.

The only way to save Hanna was a liver transplant. But Hanna wasn't healthy enough to receive one. "We had to stay in the hospital for many weeks," Melinda says. "It was a challenging time." Hanna's hepatologist noted that how healthy Hanna was before the transplant could dictate how well she would do after the transplant.

So while in the hospital, Melinda set to work. "I had to get her better so that she could be placed back on the transplant list. Advocating for someone in a hospital is hard. You can't control much, so I did the next best thing: I controlled what I could. I focused on getting my daughter better within the walls of that hospital room." Melinda made sure Hanna was rested and happy. They played games, read books and had family members come for visits. "I still remember making a balloon animal out of the hospital's disposable medical gloves and dancing it around her crib," Melinda says. "Hanna would laugh, which would make me laugh."

Hanna's health improved and she was eventually put on the liver transplant list and discharged from the hospital. Two weeks later, the family got the call that a liver from a deceased donor — Hanna's little donor angel, Melinda says — was found. They needed to get to the hospital right away.

On the drive there, Melinda remembers thinking about how the other motorists on the road, just going about their business, had no idea how monumental this day was. "None of these drivers knew that my 10-month-old daughter was about to receive a second chance at life," she says.

Several years after her successful liver transplant, Hanna is healthy and as active as any child her age. She's come a long way. "I remember the mom of another child who had a transplant telling me, 'You'll be able to relax, and it will be a lot easier,'" Melinda says. "We are down to only one medication and labs every few months, which is a stark contrast to where we started, with numerous medications, appointments and blood work.

"So, to that mom, I'd say, 'You were right.' Now we just get to watch Hanna grow and live her life to the fullest."

The day is here. A final round of testing shows the donated organ is a good match for your child, and your child is healthy enough to receive it. With the last of the pretransplant hurdles cleared, you realize it's finally happening. All the planning and preparation has led to this: another chance at life for your child.

For any parent, it's a pivotal moment that brings equal measures of hope, uncertainty and worry. No matter how much planning you've done, you're likely to feel at least somewhat frazzled or unprepared. This is understandable, given how crucial timing is with an organ transplant.

Once the organ is removed from the donor, the clock starts. Your child's transplant team will guide you regarding the amount of available time you have before the transplant. Don't forget that you've prepared for this moment, and you've got a team of experts behind you, ready to support you every step of the way.

WHAT HAPPENS DURING SURGERY

Organ transplant surgery is complex, and the time needed to complete it varies, depending on the organ being transplanted. In general, it takes several hours. Talk to your child's transplant team about how long you can expect to wait, as well as when and how you'll receive updates as the surgery progresses. If you're not certain, you also might ask where your child will be moved after the procedure. For example, your child may be moved to the pediatric intensive care unit (PICU) or another area of the hospital.

For the surgery, your child will receive general anesthesia and be placed on a breathing machine called a ventilator. If your child is receiving a heart or a lung transplant, a heart-lung bypass machine also may be used. During surgery, the machine takes over for the heart and lungs and circulates blood through the body.

Kidney transplant

For a pediatric kidney transplant, the location of the incision is dependent on the child's size. For very small children, the incision is usually in the middle of the abdomen. Larger children have an incision either on the right side or the left side of the abdomen.

The donated kidney is placed in the lower abdomen, below your child's own kidneys. In some children, the nonfunctioning kidneys may be removed. The artery and vein of the transplanted kidney are joined to an artery and vein in the pelvic area. The new kidney's ureter — the tube that links the kidney to the bladder — is connected to your child's bladder.

A tiny plastic tube called a stent may be placed in the ureter to keep it open. The stent may be linked to a small tube called a catheter that's placed in the bladder. Urine drains through the stent and catheter out of the bladder. The stent and catheter usually stay in place for a few days to a few weeks so that the bladder and ureter can heal.

Heart transplant

A transplant surgeon makes an incision in the center of your child's chest and divides your child's breastbone, also called the sternum. This approach offers the best access to your child's heart.

The transplant surgeon removes your child's damaged heart and replaces it with the donor heart. Tiny wires are inserted into the surface of your child's new heart. After surgery, these wires may be connected to a temporary pacemaker to control your child's heart rate. Sometimes after transplant surgery, the heartbeat may be too slow or erratic. Generally, the wires are removed a few days after surgery.

Drainage tubes are inserted near the chest incision. Your child may have one or two of these tubes. During healing, the tubes drain excess blood and fluids from the heart and lung area.

The breastbone is reconnected at the end of the surgery, and the incision is closed. In rare cases, a surgeon may leave the incision open at the end of heart transplant surgery. This may be needed if the surgical area is very swollen. The area is carefully covered with a dressing until the swelling goes down and the incision can be closed.

Liver transplant

A liver transplant occurs in one of three ways: The entire liver may be transplanted, a portion of a liver from a living donor may be transplanted, or a portion from a deceased donor may be transplanted. Regardless of whether your child is receiving a whole liver or part of a liver, your child's diseased liver will be removed.

During a liver transplant, a surgeon often makes an upside-down Y-shaped incision on the abdomen. Your child's diseased liver is removed through this incision and replaced with the donated liver.

LESS COMMON TRANSPLANTS

In rare cases, transplant surgery may involve other organs. A child may receive donor lungs or a donor intestine.

Lung transplant

Most lung transplants in children involve replacing both lungs. An incision is made horizontally, across the chest and beneath the breasts. The damaged lungs are removed and replaced with new organs. Your child's existing airway and blood vessels are connected to the new lungs. During surgery, your child is on a heart-lung bypass machine. The machine takes over circulation of blood and oxygen until the new lungs are functioning.

Intestinal transplant

An intestinal transplant may involve the small intestine or multiple organs in the digestive system. During an intestinal transplant, an incision is made across the abdomen. The damaged part of the intestine is removed. The donated intestine is placed and blood vessels in the new intestine are connected to your child's blood supply and the rest of the digestive system.

A temporary opening called a stoma is created in the wall of the abdomen. Stool exits through the opening and drains into an attached bag. A stoma allows the transplant team to better monitor the new intestine. It also helps give affected tissues time to heal.

Blood vessels within the new liver are connected to your child's blood vessels.

The new liver also must be connected to the bile duct so that bile can travel from the liver to the small intestine. Bile is a digestive liquid made by the liver. Sometimes a surgeon places a biliary tube inside the bile duct to help the duct function while tissues heal. The tube is generally removed 6 to 12 weeks later using minimally invasive surgery.

Small drainage tubes also may be placed in the abdomen during surgery. The tubes, which exit out either side of the abdominal wall, drain fluid and blood that may accumulate at the incision site.

IMMEDIATELY AFTER SURGERY

After transplant surgery, the focus quickly shifts to recovery and monitoring. Young transplant recipients are typically transferred to a pediatric intensive care unit, also known as the PICU. In the PICU, members of the care team monitor for signs and symptoms of organ rejection, such as fever or infection or other complications from surgery.

Blood is drawn regularly and analyzed to monitor organ function and look for signs of rejection. Imaging tests also may be performed. Depending on the child's health, time in the PICU can last for days or weeks.

Seeing your child

When you see your child for the first time after surgery, the image may be upsetting. Your child will be sedated to help with comfort. You may see a lot of tubing and monitors. These are visual reminders that your child just had major surgery and is in a fragile state right now. However, knowing more about the machines and devices may provide some comfort. Here's what you may see:

- **Breathing machine.** A breathing tube linked to a ventilator ensures that your child gets adequate oxygen until able to breathe independently. This may take a few days, depending on your child's age.
- **Monitors.** Other machines in the room track your child's vital signs, such as heart rate, oxygen levels and blood pressure.
- **Catheter.** A catheter is in your child's bladder. The attached tubing empties urine from the bladder into a bag.
- **Nose tube.** This tube, called a nasogastric tube, goes into a nostril and down to the stomach. It helps drain stomach fluid into a separate container. It also may be used to give medications to your child.
- **Intravenous (IV) bags.** Your child will receive nutrients and fluids for hydration, as well as medicine to manage pain and prevent

infection through a small tube inserted into a vein, called an IV. Through the IV your child also will receive antirejection medicine to prevent the immune system from attacking the new organ.

It may be a bit overwhelming to see your child's incision for the first time. Depending on the age of your child and the type of transplant, the incision may be large. Right after surgery, the incision — possibly closed with staples or sutures — is usually covered by a dressing. After a few days, the dressing is removed.

WHAT TO KNOW BEFORE YOU LEAVE THE HOSPITAL

To help you prepare for your child to leave the hospital, review the topics below with one of your child's nurses. Check off each item when you're confident you understand it.

Pain management
Do you know:
☐ How to use medications to relieve pain?
☐ About other pain management options?

Medications
Do you:
☐ Understand what each medication is used for?
☐ Understand the side effects of each medication?
☐ Have a schedule in place for medications? It may help to set a recurrent alarm on your smartphone as a reminder.
☐ Understand the importance of bringing your child in for blood tests?

Caring for your child
Do you know how to:
☐ Care for your child's incisions?
☐ Provide your child with the required nutrition?

If you're having trouble coping with any aspect of the transplant recovery, talk to your child's transplant team. As your child recovers, you'll play a more significant role in recovery care. It's important for you to feel comfortable and prepared for the road ahead.

NEXT STEPS

As your child recovers, there will be visible signs of progress. The breathing machine will be disconnected, and tubing removed. The

---

Maintaining contact

Do you know:

☐ When to contact your child's transplant team?

☐ How to contact your child's transplant team?

Complications

Do you understand:

☐ What rejection is?

☐ The symptoms of rejection?

☐ How to help prevent infections?

Follow-up appointments

Do you know:

☐ When your child has follow-up appointments?

☐ How to schedule follow-up appointments?

☐ The information you need to record and bring to follow-up appointments, such as your child's temperature, weight and blood pressure?

Chapter 16 goes over these points in more detail.

amount of pain medication your child is receiving will be gradually reduced. Your child will begin to move around more with help from transplant team members. Mobility is important because it can help prevent issues such as blood clots and constipation. Team members will teach your child breathing and coughing exercises to prevent pneumonia.

Once your child's condition stabilizes and the transplant team is confident that immediate risks have been managed, your child may be transferred from the PICU to a general pediatric floor. The focus remains on recovery but with less intensive monitoring. This marks a turning point and is a step closer to bringing your child home.

The transplant team will start teaching you and your child about caring for the new organ, managing medications and recognizing signs of potential complications.

Because of the risk of rejection and the complexity of post-transplant care, the transplant team will want you and your child to remain close to the transplant center for several weeks after your child is released from the hospital. Many centers, including Mayo Clinic, offer low-cost housing that's designed for families who don't live nearby.

MANAGING EMOTIONS

Children may get upset, frustrated or angry during a hospital stay. This is common. Routines are different and strangers surround them. And children in the hospital face what can seem like endless testing, and some of it can be painful. They're also not sleeping as well as they would at home.

During this time, try to follow your regular routines as best you can. Focus on soothing activities that help distract your child.

- Bring a toy or favorite blanket to help your child sleep at bedtime.
- Listen to relaxing music.
- Read or sing to your child.
- Watch funny videos or a favorite show together.
- Connect with the hospital's child life specialist for activity recommendations.

You may be experiencing a roller coaster of emotions too. Guilt, anger, relief and grief are common feelings. Social workers, therapists, chaplains and child life specialists can help you and your child with these feelings and help you cope with them.

While your presence is important for your child's recovery, taking breaks is also OK. If you're feeling tired, it's fine to sleep somewhere outside the hospital so that you can get the rest you need during this stressful time. The nursing staff will contact you if you're needed.

LOOKING AHEAD

Transplant surgery is a major step toward better health. Still, it's important to set realistic expectations for your child's recovery. The journey can be long and may include setbacks, such as complications or periods of slow progress.

The physical and emotional toll that transplant surgery can have on your child and your family is immense. Take this time to seek out counseling and support groups for help coping with changes and adjustments, including to help your child adjust to living with a transplanted organ.

Other challenges will come, and you'll learn to adjust. As your child recovers and grows, you'll establish a new normal for your family. Read more about parenting a child with a transplant in Chapter 17.

PART 4
LIFE AFTER TRANSPLANT

13

All about your medications

One of the most important aspects of life after receiving a new organ is managing your medications. Medications are key to transplant success, both in the short term and the long term. Their purpose is to keep your body from rejecting your new organ, prevent infections and treat complications that may arise after transplant surgery.

When you first leave the hospital, you'll be taking with you many medicines. Your long list of drugs will likely include several antirejection medicines. You'll also be prescribed medications to help fight infection. These generally include at least one antibiotic and one antiviral medication and perhaps an antifungal medicine. Some people need more. For example, you may need additional antibiotics if you have a donor-derived infection that requires a specific antibiotic regimen. Other medications in your initial regimen may include blood pressure or diabetes drugs and other medicines to treat or prevent potential complications.

In this chapter, we discuss several medications. It's important to know more about these drugs, their side effects and why you're taking them. Also keep in mind that the amount and type of medicine you take usually changes as time goes on. The most important drugs in your medication regimen are antirejection medications, also called immunosuppressants. These medicines are taken for life.

ANTIREJECTION MEDICINES

As the name implies, the role of antirejection medications is to make sure that your body doesn't reject your new organ. These medicines are crucial to the success of your transplant surgery. They do have side effects, however, that can range from mild to severe. Keeping your transplant team updated on how antirejection medications are affecting you can help the team create an effective drug regimen.

One side effect of antirejection medicines is that they weaken the immune system, which makes you more susceptible to colds, flu, and other bacterial, viral and fungal infections. Many infectious organisms are naturally present in the environment, and they don't affect most people with healthy immune systems. However, these organisms can sicken people whose immune systems are suppressed.

To help keep you healthy, your transplant team may recommend that you take medications such as antibiotics, antiviral medicines and, in some cases, antifungal drugs. Team members also may suggest that you take calcium and magnesium supplements because antirejection medications can reduce the level of these nutrients in your body. On the other hand, because some antirejection medications can increase potassium levels, you may need to avoid eating foods rich in potassium to keep the level of this mineral from rising too high.

The side effects of antirejection medications can seem alarming, but the risk of side effects doesn't mean that you'll experience all of them. Your susceptibility depends on your individual characteristics and circumstances. Some people experience few side effects and some experience more. Many people enjoy successful and fulfilling lives once their medications are working optimally.

Initial regimen

There are many different combinations of antirejection medications that may be used. The combination you use depends on what your care team thinks is best for you. For the several months after your surgery you'll likely be taking these medicines:

- Tacrolimus (Prograf, Astagraf XL, Envarsus XR).
- Mycophenolate mofetil (CellCept, Myhibbin).
- Prednisone.

Other antirejection medicines that may be prescribed include cyclosporine (Sandimmune), modified cyclosporine (Neoral, Gengraf), mycophenolic sodium (Myfortic), methylprednisolone (Medrol, Solu-Medrol) and azathioprine (Imuran, Azasan). You can read more about the different types of antirejection medications at the end of this chapter.

Depending on your circumstances, you may need additional medicines. If you had a heart transplant, you may be prescribed the medicine sirolimus (Rapamune) or everolimus (Afinitor, Zortress). These medicines help prevent a condition called cardiac allograft vasculopathy, in which the heart's blood vessels narrow and may become blocked.

Your transplant team may change or adjust your initial drug regimen depending on your situation and how you tolerate the drugs.

The medicines you take can produce side effects. Some can cause upset stomach or headache. They can make you hungry or cause you to gain weight. They may cause shaking, confusion or mood swings and can even lead to depression or manic episodes, in which a person experiences a drastic change in behavior that can last for a week or more. Other medicines can lead to diabetes, high blood pressure or kidney conditions and can increase your cancer risk. Your transplant team works with you to optimize your medications for your overall health.

If you develop diabetes, high blood pressure, high cholesterol or other concerning conditions, more medicines may be added to your regimen to treat these conditions. For example, you may need blood pressure medication or insulin shots. If you experience mood swings or depression, you may be prescribed antidepressants. You can read more about medications to treat side effects later in this chapter.

It's important to understand that the chances of organ rejection are highest the first year after surgery. When you first start anti-rejection medications, you'll be taking high doses. Side effects are likely to be most challenging during this initial period and generally get better with time.

Gradually, your doses will be reduced. You also may be able to stop taking some of the medicines. For example, most people can stop taking steroids, such as prednisone, within four months after surgery. As a result, some side effects, including diabetes, tend to disappear, and others become less severe. In addition, depending on the type of transplant you receive, you may not need antibiotics after a year, and you also may no longer need blood pressure medication. While the first few months after surgery may feel strenuous and exhausting, your health, mood and overall sense of well-being should improve over time.

Checkups

During the first year after your transplant, you'll need to return to the medical center where you had your surgery every few months for checkups. After that you'll likely come back once or twice a year.

Once you're home, you can go back to seeing your local healthcare team for general health issues. For example, if you develop a sinus infection a year after your surgery, you won't need to travel all the way to your transplant hospital for a prescription. A medical professional at your local clinic can help you.

Be sure everyone who cares for you, including the pharmacists you see, knows about the medications you're taking as well as any restrictions you must follow. This is important because some medications can affect how your antirejection medicines work. If you're given a new prescription and you're not sure about it, contact your transplant team before taking it.

Medicines and foods to avoid

Certain medicines that you can purchase without a prescription may interact with your antirejection medications. These include products such as aspirin, ibuprofen (Advil, Motrin IB, others) and naproxen sodium (Aleve). Don't take these medicines unless your transplant team tells you that you can. Instead, take acetaminophen (Tylenol, others) for minor pain such as headaches.

But don't take acetaminophen for a fever unless your transplant team tells you it's OK. If you have a fever, your transplant team may want to check for an infection. You should have necessary tests before taking any medication for fever, such as acetaminophen.

Common acid-reducing medicines that calm heartburn and upset stomach and are available without a prescription also can interfere with your antirejection medications. These medicines include magnesium antacids (Phillips' Milk of Magnesia), other antacids containing magnesium (Mylanta, Maalox) and cimetidine (Tagamet HB). Don't use these products unless approved by your transplant team.

Vitamins, supplements and probiotics can affect how your antirejection medications work too. As a rule, avoid taking these products unless your transplant team gives you a go-ahead.

Lastly, some foods and drinks may interfere with antirejection medications. For example, grapefruit, pomegranates, Seville oranges and similar types of citrus fruits can cause levels of the medications tacrolimus, sirolimus and cyclosporine to rise too high. Avoid eating these fruits as well as any preserves, marmalades, juices, smoothies or soft drinks that may contain them. Ask about the ingredients

DO NOT TAKE

- Ibuprofen (Advil, Motrin IB, others) or naproxen sodium (Aleve).
- Aspirin, unless prescribed by your transplant team.
- Vitamins, unless prescribed by your transplant team.
- Herbal supplements.
- Probiotic supplements.
- Cimetidine (Tagamet HB).
- Magnesium antacids (Phillips' Milk of Magnesia) or other antacids that contain magnesium (Mylanta, Maalox).

when ordering drinks and read ingredient labels when buying items at the store.

MEDICATIONS TO TREAT SIDE EFFECTS

Antirejection medications can cause side effects, especially in the first few months after transplant surgery when the medications are taken in higher doses. If you experience side effects, such as diabetes or high blood pressure, you may need to take other medicines to manage your symptoms.

To lower blood sugar

Some antirejection medications, such as prednisone, can increase blood sugar levels. You may need to check your blood sugar at home to make sure it isn't getting too high. If your blood sugar becomes elevated, your transplant team may prescribe insulin shots or other medicines taken by mouth to lower it to a healthy level.

To lower blood pressure

Some antirejection medications can raise your blood pressure. Again, you may need to regularly check your blood pressure at home. If it's too high, you may need to take medicines to lower it. Different types of blood pressure medications have different side effects, so your transplant team will help you find what works best in your case.

To treat bacterial infections

Antibiotics prevent or treat infections caused by bacteria. They aren't effective for viral infections, such as a common cold or the flu. Some antibiotics, such as the medicines erythromycin and clarithromycin, can interfere with antirejection medication levels.

If your transplant team prescribes an antibiotic, take it as long as recommended. If a medical professional at home prescribes an antibiotic, make sure that person is aware of all the medications you're taking, especially your antirejection medications. If there's a concern about a possible interaction with your medications, contact your transplant team to make sure you can safely take the antibiotic.

WHAT TO TAKE

Symptom	Medication

Pain	• Acetaminophen (Tylenol, others)
	
	  ◦ Regular-strength acetaminophen: 325 mg
	  ◦ Extra-strength acetaminophen: 500 mg
	
	You may take a maximum of 3,000 mg in a 24-hour period. Make sure to read the labels of your other medications because they also may contain acetaminophen. Be careful not to exceed this dose.

Allergies	• Diphenhydramine (Benadryl) • Cetirizine (Zyrtec) • Loratadine (Claritin, Alavert)
Cough, congestion	• Plain guaifenesin (Mucinex, Robitussin Mucus Plus Chest Congestion)
Constipation	• Senna, bisacodyl (Dulcolax, Correctol, others) • Polyethylene glycol 3350 (Miralax) • Docusate sodium (Colace) • Psyllium (Metamucil, Konsyl, others) with plenty of water • Methylcellulose (Citrucel) with plenty of water • Wheat dextrin (Benefiber) with plenty of water

Consult with a medical professional before taking these medications to determine which options are best for you.

To treat viral infections

Antiviral medications prevent or treat infections caused by the herpes virus. These viruses include cytomegalovirus (CMV) and Epstein-Barr virus. Also in this family are viruses that cause chickenpox and shingles, also known as herpes zoster, and cold sores, also called herpes simplex. If your transplant team prescribes an antiviral, don't stop taking it until you're told you no longer need it. If a medical professional at home prescribes an antiviral, check with your transplant team before taking it.

To treat fungal infections

Antifungal medications prevent or treat fungal infections on your skin or in your mouth, lungs, digestive tract or other parts of your body. Antifungal drugs may affect levels of your antirejection medications. As a result, the amount of antirejection medication you take may need to be adjusted.

If your transplant team prescribes an antifungal, don't stop taking it until you're told you no longer need it. If a healthcare professional at home prescribes an antifungal, you may need to contact your transplant team to adjust the amount of your antirejection medication. Make sure the transplant team is also aware when you stop taking antifungal medications. Your antirejection medication may need to be readjusted. This may require frequent blood checks to confirm that you're receiving the right amounts of the drugs.

MANAGING MEDICATION REGIMENS

It's important that you understand when and how to take your transplant medications. If you have questions, ask your transplant team. They're there to assist you. In addition, here are a few tips to help you keep your medicine regimen organized.

Track your medications

Keep a list of the medicines you're currently taking, along with their generic and brand names, the prescribed dose, and what time of day to take them. You can do this using a notebook or journal. Or you might use a digital app on your phone or an electronic spreadsheet on your computer. Often, digital apps also notify you when to take the medication and they keep a history of what you've taken in the past.

Always bring a list of your medications to all medical appointments and when getting prescriptions from a pharmacist so they know what you're taking.

Pay attention to strengths
Some medications may be prescribed in different strengths. For example, for certain medications you may be given both 1-milligram and 5-milligram tablets. You may need to combine them to equal the dosage you're prescribed. If you have questions about taking medications of different strengths, talk with your transplant team or your pharmacist.

Take your medicines as directed
Some of your transplant medicines may come as large capsules or tablets. They may be hard to swallow, but they should be taken whole and not crushed, cut or split. If you aren't able to swallow your medicines, speak with your transplant team so they can come up with a safe and efficient alternative.

If you miss your medication
Life after transplant surgery can get complex. There may come a moment when you miss a medication dose. You also may get sick and throw up shortly after taking your medications, which means that your body didn't have a chance to absorb the medicine. If that happens, you may or may not need another dose. Talk with your transplant team and ask what to do in such situations.

Store your pills correctly
Keep your pills in their original containers. Store pills inside their closed containers at room temperature. Keep pills away from heat, moisture and direct sunlight. Don't store medications in the bathroom, above the refrigerator or near a sink because heat and moisture from your shower, bath, sink or refrigerator motor may damage your medicine. The medicines can become less potent, or they may go bad before the expiration date.

Store your liquids correctly

Keep liquid medicines in their original containers. Some liquids need to be refrigerated. Others should be stored at room temperature. Talk with your pharmacist about how to store your liquid medications. If you can keep them at room temperature, don't store them in the bathroom to avoid damaging them.

Plan ahead for refills

Ask your insurance company when you can refill your prescriptions. Many companies let you refill at least one week before you run out of medications. Others may let you refill sooner. Plan ahead so you don't run out of medications. If you're going to be away from home for a certain period of time, make sure you have enough medicine with you.

Use a single pharmacy

Try to use the same pharmacy so your pharmacist knows what you're taking and can check your medications for interactions. If you use more than one pharmacy, this important safety check may not happen. If your transplant team says it's OK to take certain herbs, supplements or other nonprescription products, make sure to tell your pharmacist what you're using so the pharmacist can check for any interactions.

Make sure you have the right medicines

When refilling your medications, check your refills before you leave the pharmacy. If your medications look different, ask the pharmacist if you've been given the right ones. Once you leave the pharmacy, you generally can't return your medications.

If you use a mail-order pharmacy, talk with the pharmacist about how important it is that you get the exact medications you've been prescribed. Request that staff members at your mail-order pharmacy inform you if they substitute a medication with a similar drug before they mail your medicine. Depending on your insurance coverage, pharmacies may substitute brand-name medications with generics. In many cases, generics are acceptable, but sometimes they may not be. If your pharmacy substitutes your medication with generics, contact your transplant team. Always tell your transplant team about any medication substitutions.

Check expiration dates
Expired medicines may not work as they're supposed to. Instead of helping you, they may be harmful. If your medicines expire, don't use them. Get a new refill instead. Talk with your pharmacist about how to dispose of medications properly.

ANTIREJECTION MEDICATIONS AT A GLANCE
Here's additional information on specific antirejection medicines, what they do, and common side effects associated with them.

Prednisone and methylprednisolone (Medrol, Solu-Medrol)
Prednisone is a corticosteroid drug. It suppresses your immune system's overall response and robustness. Methylprednisolone is a similar medication but is more potent. Both medications can produce many side effects, which may range from mild to severe:
- Increased appetite.
- Weight gain.
- Upset stomach.
- Muscle cramps, pain or weakness.
- Changes in mood.
- Difficulty sleeping.
- Acne.
- Thin, shiny skin.
- Rounding of your face.
- Streaks on abdominal skin.
- High blood sugar.
- High blood pressure.
- Diabetes.
- Swelling in your legs.
- Cataracts.
- Reduced bone mass.
- Bone injury.

Mycophenolate mofetil (CellCept, Myhibbin), mycophenolic sodium (Myfortic)

These medications reduce the formation of a type of white blood cell called a lymphocyte that helps the body's immune system fight infection and disease. In addition to increasing your risk of infection and illness, this type of medication can have the following side effects:

- Nausea or vomiting.
- Diarrhea or constipation.
- High blood sugar.
- Blood pressure changes.
- Increased heart rate.
- Headache.
- Dizziness.
- Shakiness.
- Swelling of the lower legs and feet.
- Difficulty sleeping.

If you're taking this type of drug, don't take antacid medications containing magnesium to relieve heartburn, acid indigestion or an upset stomach. They may interfere with how your body uses the antirejection medication.

It's also important to prevent pregnancy, as the medications can harm an unborn baby, also called a fetus. Read more about pregnancy after transplant surgery on pages 232-233.

Tacrolimus (Prograf, Astagraf XL, Envarsus XR)

Tacrolimus suppresses the production and spread of specialized white blood cells called T lymphocytes that are responsible for causing rejection. Because this reduces your immune defense, the medication increases your risk of infection and illness. Tacrolimus also may cause a variety of side effects that may range from mild to severe:

- Headache.
- Sinus congestion.
- Hair thinning or hair loss.
- Stomach pain.
- Diarrhea or constipation.
- Shakiness.

MEDICINES, FOODS AND BEVERAGES THAT DON'T MIX

Some foods and beverages can affect how your body uses the medications tacrolimus (Prograf, Astagraf XL, Envarsus XR), sirolimus (Rapamune) and cyclosporine (Sandimmune). For example, certain types of citrus and other fruit can make the levels of these medications rise too high.

If you take tacrolimus, sirolimus and cyclosporine, don't eat:
- Grapefruit.
- Seville oranges, also called Spanish, sour or bitter oranges. They're often found in orange marmalade.
- Pomelos, a fruit similar to grapefruit.
- Pomegranates.

Also avoid drinking soft drinks, juice blends, iced tea or smoothies that contain juices or extracts from these fruits. And you must avoid food or candy that has the same ingredients.

It's OK to eat clementines but limit them to no more than six a day. Other types of oranges also are safe to eat.

- High blood pressure.
- Increased blood sugar levels.
- Increased potassium levels.
- Kidney conditions.

Sirolimus (Rapamune)

Sirolimus also suppresses the activation and spread of T lymphocytes, and it inhibits production of antibodies. Antibodies are proteins that help the body's immune system fight off foreign substances, including viruses and bacteria. Side effects may include the following:
- Skin rash.
- Diarrhea.
- Mouth sores.

- Swelling in your legs.
- Longer time for wounds to heal.
- Anemia due to low red blood cell counts.
- Lung conditions.
- Increased triglycerides and cholesterol in blood.

Sirolimus also shouldn't be taken during pregnancy due to risks to the unborn child.

Cyclosporine (Sandimmune) and modified cyclosporine (Neoral, Gengraf)

Cyclosporine also reduces the activity of the immune system's T lymphocytes similar to sirolimus. Cyclosporine may produce the following side effects:
- Extra hair growth.
- Gum thickening.
- Leg cramps.
- Nausea.
- High blood pressure.
- Increased cholesterol.
- High blood sugar.
- High potassium.
- Kidney conditions.

Azathioprine (Imuran, Azasan)

This medication also works by decreasing the production and spread of specialized immune system cells, suppressing immune system activity. Side effects may include the following:
- Nausea or vomiting.
- Blood in stool or urine.
- Lower back or side pain.
- Hoarseness and cough.
- Tiny spots on skin.
- Mouth or lip sores or ulcers.
- Fatigue.
- Weakness and muscle pain.
- Unusual bruising.

FOR CAREGIVERS: TIPS FOR MANAGING MEDICATIONS

Managing your loved one's medications may feel overwhelming, particularly during the early phase of recovery when both you and the person you care for are still adjusting to a new normal. For the first few months after surgery, the person in your care may feel tired, anxious, forgetful or confused — in large part due to the side effects of the medications they're taking. That's where your help is needed.

You can help by organizing your loved one's prescription bottles in a useful way or by creating schedules and checklists of what to take and when. You also can help by taking notes during appointments and keeping track of the doses, frequencies and expiration dates of the various prescriptions. Another way to help is by making sure the person in your care stays away from nonprescription medicines that aren't safe to take. And you can help by staying on top of medication refills and communicating with the pharmacists filling the prescriptions.

In addition, keep a close eye on the foods and beverages that your loved one is consuming to make sure that they don't contain ingredients that are prohibited. For example, to keep antirejection medications working properly, it's important for a person taking immunosuppressants to avoid grapefruit, pomegranate, Seville oranges and similar types of citrus fruits. These ingredients are commonly found in soft drinks, juices, preserves, marmalades and other items. Check ingredient labels to make sure that your loved one's food and drinks don't contain these ingredients.

With time, medication management should become easier. As your loved one's health improves, some medications may no longer be needed and others can be taken at lower doses. This may reduce some side effects, helping the person in your care to feel better. Eventually, the daily medication routine will likely become second nature to you and your loved one.

14

Adjusting to a new normal

Recovering from transplant surgery can bring feelings of both excitement and anxiety. You may feel like you're starting a new life, but at the same time you may be very nervous about what lies ahead. These feelings are common. Many people who receive a transplant experience a host of emotions as they leave the hospital.

SHORT-TERM RECOVERY
Keep in mind that if you live far from your transplant center, you likely won't go home right away. You'll stay near the hospital for a few weeks to a few months to make sure that your new organ is doing well. How long you remain in temporary housing depends on how quickly your health and mobility are improving and, even more so, on the type of transplant you received.

These are approximate durations for how long you'll likely need to stay close to your transplant center, based on organ type.

- Kidney transplant: 3 to 4 weeks.
- Kidney-pancreas transplant: 4 to 6 weeks.
- Liver transplant: 4 to 6 weeks.
- Heart transplant: 2 to 3 months.
- Lung transplant: 3 to 4 months.

During your initial recovery period, expect to return to the transplant center several times a week for blood tests, biopsies, physical therapy, medication adjustments and other appointments to optimize your health and recovery. During this time, you also may start

SIGNS AND SYMPTOMS OF REJECTION

Rejection can happen at any time. However, it's more common within the first year after a transplant. In the early stages of rejection, you may feel fine. However, if you start having the following symptoms, contact your transplant team right away.
- Feeling very tired or weak.
- A heartbeat that is unusually fast or feels like it skips some beats.
- Shortness of breath.
- Swelling in your hands, feet or ankles.
- Weight change of 3 to 5 pounds or more over two days.
- Flu-like aches and pains.
- Blood pressure that is significantly lower than your usual blood pressure.

If your transplant team thinks you may be experiencing a rejection episode, you may need to return to the transplant center for tests, including a biopsy of your transplanted organ. Your transplant team also may need to adjust your antirejection medication.

managing your own medications and doing more of your own daily care instead of relying on your caregiver.

Your care team likely will provide helpful instructions for managing your overall health and well-being in the months and years ahead, including information on worrisome signs and symptoms to watch for. You can read more about self-care in the next chapter.

You shouldn't drive for at least 2 to 6 weeks after surgery, especially if you're taking pain medications, so you'll need to rely on your caregiver to get you to and from your appointments. It's also important that you avoid lifting anything heavier than 10 pounds — about the weight of a gallon of milk — for at least eight weeks after surgery. This provides adequate time for your incisions to heal properly.

If you're a gardener, wait at least six months before you start digging in the dirt again. Soil can contain microorganisms that may cause infections. When you do get back to gardening, wear gloves and a mask.

GOING HOME

When your transplant team feels good about your progress, you can leave your temporary housing and go home. If home is a distance away, you may need to make some special arrangements to travel safely. If you'll be flying home, you or your caregiver may want to call the airline and request a wheelchair or order special meals, if appropriate.

Transporting your medications

If you're flying home, make sure to put all your medications into your carry-on bag. This prevents you from losing them if your checked luggage gets left behind, and it gives you easy access to the medications, if you need to take them.

Keep your medications in their original bottles or containers. If your medication comes in a liquid form, you should be able to get it through airport security even if it exceeds the allowable 3.4-fluid-ounce size. But it's a good idea to ask your transplant team for a note.

If you're traveling home by car, don't put your medications where they could become too hot or too cold.

Preventing blood clots

When you sit for several hours during a long flight or a car ride, your risk of developing blood clots in your legs increases. This is especially true after surgery. To lower that risk during a flight, take a walk up and down the airplane aisle once every hour or so.

If you're traveling by car, make stops every few hours and walk around the car a time or two. While sitting in the car or on the plane, move your feet and legs when you can: Flex your feet. Rotate your ankles. Raise your toes up and down.

Ask your transplant team whether you should wear compression stockings to help blood circulation in your legs. Blood clots tend to form when you don't have enough fluids in your body, called dehydration. So make sure to drink plenty of fluids before and during travel.

When you get home

Once back home, you'll generally see your local healthcare team for most of your health needs. Make sure all local medical professionals you see are aware of the medications you're taking. And make sure they know how to contact your transplant team if a concerning situation arises. During the first year after your surgery, you'll usually need to return to the transplant center a few times for checkups, tests and biopsies. But if all goes well in the years that follow, you may only need to return once or twice a year.

Because the antirejection medications you're taking interfere with your immune system's ability to fight germs and potential infections, it's important that you continue to take precautions to avoid getting sick when you get home. Practice good hygiene and take other measures to stay healthy. These measures include not being around people who are sick, washing your hands with soap immediately and thoroughly after a cut or scrape, and following safety rules when handling or preparing food or caring for pets.

Other precautions

You may want to wear a medical ID bracelet or necklace. A medical ID bracelet or necklace holds your health information in case you cannot talk during a medical emergency. In your case, the necklace or bracelet can say that you've had a transplant and list the medications you're taking as well as allergies and other conditions you have. If you'd like such an item, ask your transplant team how to obtain one.

FOOD SAFETY

Food poisoning can happen to anyone, but for people taking anti-rejection medications, the risk is greater, and the illness can be more troubling.

Because your immune system is suppressed, you're more susceptible to infections such as food poisoning. You also may need longer to recover from such illnesses. In addition, throwing up and having diarrhea can affect how much your body is able to absorb your anti-rejection medication, if at all. This can place you at risk of rejecting your new organ.

That's why handling food properly is so important. Here are some strategies to live by.

Shopping

Food safety begins at the supermarket. If you observe a typical supermarket scene, you'll likely notice that many shoppers simply stack their items in the carts in the order they pick them up. It's not uncommon to see a package of pork chops resting on a carton of raspberries, or a carton of ice cream sitting atop a salmon fillet.

All uncooked meat, poultry and seafood harbor bacteria, such as listeria or salmonella, or parasites. And it's not uncommon for these microorganisms to settle on packaging while raw foods are being cut and wrapped. Even when the packages appear clean, a few smears can deposit a myriad of such organisms on package surfaces.

When these packages touch other food items in the cart — fresh produce, cereal boxes or jam jars — the germs transfer onto them. This is called cross-contamination. And while fruit and vegetables are usually washed before eating, cereal boxes and jam jars generally aren't.

For people whose immune systems aren't suppressed, this type of cross-contamination usually doesn't pose a serious threat. Even if they consume some of the germs that are transferred from one food item to another, their immune systems will usually wipe out the bugs before they cause serious harm.

People who take antirejection medicines generally don't have this type of protection and need to take extra precautions. When food shopping, it's important to separate uncooked foods such as meats, poultry, sausages, seafood and eggs from ready-to-eat items. It's also a good idea to double-bag all uncooked food to create an extra layer of protection. When checking out, make sure all uncooked food, including eggs, is placed into a separate bag.

Also, when purchasing fruit juice, milk, cheese and other dairy products, make sure you select pasteurized options. Pasteurized means that the foods have been heated to a certain temperature to kill any bacteria that may naturally lurk inside. For example, unpasteurized milk may contain organisms such as campylobacter, *Escherichia* (*E.*) *coli*, listeria or salmonella. Therefore, make sure the milk you buy is labeled as pasteurized.

Cheeses made from unpasteurized milk may contain these microorganisms too. Soft cheeses such as brie, feta, Camembert, Roquefort, queso blanco and queso fresco are often made from unpasteurized milk, so it's best to avoid them. With all cheeses, check that they're made from pasteurized milk.

There are other foods to be aware of. Products such as Caesar salad dressing, hollandaise sauce and eggnog may contain uncooked eggs, which can harbor salmonella. These items are best avoided as well. Mayonnaise is usually made with pasteurized eggs, but it's a good idea to check the label. Lastly, always adhere to the expiration dates and use-by dates on the items you buy.

Cooking

To prevent cross-contamination at home, keep uncooked foods separate from ready-to-eat foods. Here are some tips to consider:

Thawing

When thawing raw or cooked meat, poultry or other perishables, avoid doing it at room temperature, such as on kitchen countertops, where various bacteria may be present. Instead, thaw food in the refrigerator, in cold water or in the microwave. If you use the microwave, cook the food immediately after it's defrosted.

It's important to cook food thoroughly to prevent illness. Here's a guide to follow:

- **Poultry.** Cook all poultry, including ground chicken and turkey, to 165 degrees Fahrenheit.
- **Beef, lamb, pork, veal.** Cook all raw beef, lamb, pork and veal steaks, roasts, and chops to 145 degrees Fahrenheit with a three-minute rest time after removal from the heat source.
- **Ground meat.** Cook ground meats such as beef and pork to at least 160 degrees Fahrenheit.
- **Ham.** Reheat fully cooked ham that was packaged at a USDA-inspected plant to 140 degrees Fahrenheit. If the product was repackaged at another location or if you're using leftover cooked ham, heat it to 165 degrees Fahrenheit.
- **Seafood.** Cook seafood to 145 degrees Fahrenheit. When preparing shrimp, lobster or crab, cook until the shells turn red and the flesh is pearly opaque. Cook clams, mussels and oysters until the shells open. Discard shellfish that don't open.
- **Eggs.** Cook eggs until the yolks and whites are firm. Don't eat any food containing raw eggs, such as homemade hollandaise sauce or raw cookie dough. Use only recipes in which the egg ingredients are heated to 160 degrees Fahrenheit.
- **Sauces, gravies and soups.** When reheating sauces, soups or gravy, bring them to a boil.
- **Leftovers.** Heat other leftovers to 165 degrees Fahrenheit.

Using a food thermometer, check the food's internal temperature in more than one location.

Preparing

Have one cutting board that you use only for raw foods such as meat, poultry and seafood. Use a different one for ready-to-eat foods, such as bread, fresh fruits and vegetables, and cooked meat.

After chopping or cutting one food item, wash all used utensils with soap and water before moving to the next item. Wash all cutting surfaces thoroughly with soap and water.

Don't place cooked meats, poultry, seafood or eggs onto a plate that previously held raw items. If you must use the same plate, wash it thoroughly with hot, soapy water and dry it with a clean towel before reloading it. If you marinate raw foods, don't use the marinades as dressings unless you boil them first.

Heating

To make sure meats and other raw proteins are free of harmful bacteria, cook them fully to the right temperatures. Use a food thermometer to check the food's internal temperature. Check in several places to make sure your turkey, meatloaf or lamb roast is cooked evenly all the way through.

Cleaning up

Keeping your kitchen clean is essential. Bacteria can easily spread throughout the kitchen, getting onto countertops, cutting boards and utensils and ultimately into your food. Clean and sanitize kitchen counters often. Wash utensils and cutting boards in a dishwasher if possible.

Use disposable paper towels to clean kitchen surfaces. If you're using cloth towels, wash them frequently using the hot cycle of the washing machine. Clean the lids of canned goods before opening them just in case germs have settled there.

Storing food

The refrigerator and freezer are your friends. Cold temperatures slow bacterial growth. With that in mind, here are some tips for safely storing food.

- Remember to put all perishable items in the refrigerator or freezer shortly after you bring them home. In the refrigerator, keep meat

How do you know if your cold cuts or leftovers are still safe to eat? You may not know. Foodborne microorganisms can be hard to detect. And looking at, smelling or tasting food doesn't always tell you whether it's safe. Your cold cuts may look just fine, but listeria, salmonella or campylobacter may already be multiplying inside.

Don't taste questionable food to determine whether it's good to eat. Even small amounts of germs or other microbes can make you sick. To be safe, remember: When in doubt, throw it out.

and fish packages separate from produce, butter, cream cheese, salads or preserves.

- Refrigerate or freeze meat, poultry, eggs, seafood, and other items that can spoil within two hours of cooking or purchasing them. If the outside temperature is above 90 degrees Fahrenheit, refrigerate within one hour.
- Split large amounts of food into smaller or shallower containers so the food chills faster in the refrigerator.
- Make sure to reheat leftovers to the right temperature (see page 203). Reheat hot dogs, cold cuts, other deli-style meats and poultry as well as smoked seafood to 165 degrees Fahrenheit.

PET SAFETY

If you have pets, you'll need to follow a few precautions to minimize your risk of infection. Pets are wonderful companions who often bring considerable joy to life. However, they can carry bacteria, viruses, parasites and fungi that don't affect them but may spread to people through animal saliva or waste or through a bite or scratch.

These microorganisms can sicken people who have weakened immune systems. Taking a few precautions with your pets can minimize your risk of disease.

At the vet
- Ask your veterinarian to check all your pets for infectious diseases.
- Have your cat checked for *Bartonella henselae*, the organism responsible for cat scratch disease. Also have the vet check for the feline leukemia and feline immunodeficiency viruses. While these viruses don't bother humans, they weaken cats' immune systems, making cats more susceptible to infections with other germs that may spread to humans.
- Keep your pets' vaccinations current.
- Have your pets surgically spayed or neutered. Neutered animals are less likely to roam, and therefore less likely to get diseases.
- Seek veterinary care if your pet has diarrhea, is coughing and sneezing, has decreased appetite, or has lost weight.

Everyday care
- Keep your pets clean and healthy.
- Wash your hands after having contact with a pet or any other animal.
- If you plan to adopt a pet, choose one that's at least one year old. Kittens and puppies are more likely to scratch, bite and pass on their germs to you.
- If you're scratched or bitten, wash the area with soap and water and watch for signs of infection. Contact your local healthcare team if you see any signs of infection.
- Wear gloves when you trim a pet's nails, do other pet grooming or clean an aquarium. Keep your pet's nails short.
- Feed your pet only commercially prepared food and treats. Don't let them catch or eat wild animals, such as mice or birds. Wild animals can carry diseases that can affect your pets and you.
- Some bacterial and viral infections are spread by fleas and ticks, which dogs and cats may get. To prevent flea or tick infestations, use flea preventatives and choose permethrin-treated bedding for your pets.

Things to avoid
- Don't let your pet drink from the toilet. Several infections can happen this way.

- Avoid changing your cat's litter box yourself. Have someone else do it. If you have no one to help you, wear gloves and a mask, and wash your hands thoroughly after you're done.
- Don't let your pets roam on their own outside. This helps minimize their contact with wild animals and associated infections.
- Avoid putting your dog in a boarding kennel or similar facility. Dogs can develop a condition called kennel cough while in a kennel that can cause illness in people with weakened immune systems.
- Avoid keeping pet birds, rodents, amphibians or reptiles because they may carry salmonella.

MINIMIZING INFECTIONS

When out in public it can be difficult to not get sick. But there are a few things that you can do to reduce your risk. One of them is to keep your vaccinations up to date. Another is to avoid being around people who are sick. There are times you also may want to wear a face mask. And remember to wash your hands frequently with soap and water. Always wash your hands after using the bathroom or getting a scrape or cut and before handling your medication.

Vaccinations

Work with your local healthcare team to stay current on your vaccinations, including seasonal shots such as the flu and COVID-19 vaccines.

An important point: After transplant surgery, make sure that the vaccines you receive don't contain a live virus. Because your immune system is suppressed, a live virus can make you sick. Get your flu vaccine as a shot, not as a nasal mist. The nasal mist contains a live virus.

People living in your home and others you're frequently around also should get the vaccine as a shot, not as a nasal mist, so they won't pass the live virus on to you.

Several other vaccines contain live viruses. Discuss with your transplant team the need for vaccines for polio, measles, mumps, rubella, shingles and chickenpox. Also, stay away from people who receive live vaccines for 10 days after their vaccinations.

Infections

Because your immune system is weakened, an infection can become a serious matter. Following are some common infections that can develop after a transplant. Your transplant team will carefully watch for signs and symptoms of these illnesses. You also may have blood tests to monitor for such infections.

Contact your transplant team promptly if you notice any signs and symptoms of an infection (see page 210).

Cytomegalovirus (CMV)

This virus is spread through close contact with an infected person or from contact with body fluids, such as saliva or nasal discharge. Once you get CMV, it becomes dormant in your body and may not cause symptoms for a long time.

However, a dormant virus can reactivate, years later, and cause another infection. Because your immune system is weakened, you're at an increased risk of this occurring. After your surgery, your transplant team may put you on certain antiviral medications to prevent reactivation. CMV may lead to rejection of your transplanted organ or become life-threatening, but it can be treated with antiviral medications. You'll learn about symptoms to watch for to catch the infection early if reactivation does occur.

Epstein-Barr virus (EBV)

This virus is spread by close contact with another person's saliva. EBV causes infectious mononucleosis, often called mono. Like getting CMV, once you get EBV, it becomes dormant in your body and can reactivate. In transplant recipients, EBV infection can be severe and can lead to post-transplant lymphoproliferative disease, also called lymphoma. This is a type of immune system cancer that must be treated.

BK virus

This virus is very common, and many people get it in childhood. It stays dormant in the urinary system but can reactivate once you start taking antirejection medications. In some people, the virus can damage a transplanted kidney. BK virus infection can be successfully treated, especially when found early.

WHEN A TRANSPLANT FAILS

Most transplants are successful. Some, however, result in complications. Sometimes these complications can be remediated and sometimes they can't. When they can't, the organ fails — and you'll need another transplant.

Transplants are complex medical procedures. This means that things may happen that are beyond a patient's or the transplant team's control. Blood clots can develop inside a transplanted organ, interfering with the flow of oxygen and damaging the organ. An infection can take hold within a transplanted organ, which can cause a life-threatening condition known as sepsis.

Sometimes, chronic rejection may occur, slowly damaging the organ. In the case of chronic rejection, if caught early enough, the transplant team may be able to take action to reverse the rejection and prevent the need for another transplant.

No one wants to repeat the transplant process. But if it happens to you, try to stay strong and keep the faith. Some people go through a transplant procedure more than once and arrive at a happy ending.

Shingles
This condition results from the same virus that causes chickenpox. It happens when the virus reactivates in the body years later. The first signs may be pain, itching and tingling in an area of skin on one side of your body or face. A painful blistering rash then appears in the same area. If you get shingles, early diagnosis is important so it can be treated with antiviral medications.

Pneumonia
An infection that occurs in your lungs, pneumonia may result from viruses, bacteria or fungi. The type of treatment you receive depends on your specific infection.

WHEN TO CALL

It may not always be easy to know if you're getting sick. Or you may not be sure if the signs and symptoms you're experiencing are something serious or nothing at all. The important thing to remember is that it's better to be safe than sorry. If you're not sure what's happening, err on the side of caution and contact your transplant team.

Call the team immediately if you:

- Have a steady rise or fall in your blood pressure readings.
- Notice a weight gain of 3 pounds or more from the previous morning.
- Have any blood in your urine or stool or bleeding from another source that won't stop.
- Have nausea or vomiting or cannot keep down your medications.
- Are urinating less, have foul-smelling urine, or feel pain or burning when urinating.
- Have a temperature above 101 degrees Fahrenheit.
- Have difficulty breathing.
- Have a cough with green or yellow mucus.
- Have pus, swelling, hardness or warmth around your transplant incision.
- Are experiencing headaches, tremors or shaky hands.
- Experience more than one episode of watery diarrhea.
- Are experiencing worsening medication side effects.
- Haven't passed stool for three days, especially if you're taking narcotic pain medications, such as oxycodone (Oxycontin, Roxicodone, others).
- Have flu-like symptoms such as chills, nausea, throwing up, dizziness, body aches or severe weakness.
- Forget or aren't able to take your medication at a scheduled time for any reason.

FOR CAREGIVERS: SETTLING IN

Like your loved one, you may be thrilled and happy to be going home. You may have a sense of relief that the hardest part of the transplant experience is over. You may even feel hope that the journey is nearing its end.

DOS AND DON'TS OF HOME SELF-CARE

Do:

- Take your temperature twice a day. A temperature below 101 degrees Fahrenheit is generally considered to be within the standard range. The further you get from your transplant date, the less frequently this must be done.
- Take your blood pressure twice each day. You generally want to see blood pressures between 100/60 and 130/90. You can take your blood pressure less frequently the farther you are from your transplant date.
- Weigh yourself once a day in the morning after you use the restroom and record your weight.
- Drink plenty of fluids, up to a gallon a day unless otherwise advised.
- Keep a current medication list with you so that you can show it to medical personnel, including dentists and pharmacists.
- Always keep on hand a seven-day supply of your medications. Get your refills early so you don't run out.
- Attend all follow-up appointments. Skipping follow-ups can lead to preventable complications or even life-threatening situations.

Don't:

- Stop taking your medications or make changes to the dose unless your transplant team tells you to do so. Talk to your transplant team if you are experiencing any side effects.
- Eat grapefruit, Seville oranges or pomegranates, as they may interfere with the levels of antirejection medications in your blood.
- Drink any juices or other beverages that contain these fruits.
- Take any new prescription — or any vitamins, minerals and other nonprescription products — before checking with your transplant team.

Jill's story

When Jill was told that her husband needed a liver transplant, she wasn't ready for the news. Patrick had just battled through a life-threatening illness and was recovering, so she thought they were over the hump. Hearing that he now needed to undergo transplant surgery was hard to comprehend.

Talking to her friends and family helped her come to terms with it. "You need to verbalize what's happening so that you yourself can come to a reality," she says. "I think talking about it makes people realize how serious the situation is and helps them come to grips with what their role in the situation is." Soon, however, she realized that keeping every person in her various social circles up to date on every development was exhausting, so she narrowed down her communications to only a few dedicated individuals. "I spoke to two people, and I let them do the chain of communication however they wanted to keep other people in the loop."

Having cared for her husband and for her parents when they got older, Jill was an experienced caregiver. But the transplant journey required a different level of care: being on call 24-7 and being super organized. Keeping track of Patrick's medications was challenging because the doses changed often — sometimes twice or even three times a week. To avoid constantly putting medicines together and separating them to adjust to the new doses, Jill prepared enough doses to last to the next appointment only. "I tried to break everything down into the smallest steps so that I didn't get overwhelmed by the process," she says.

To ensure that Patrick took his medications every morning and evening at the same time, Jill set alarms on her cell phone. "At some point, he also had to take magnesium at noon, so that alarm went off and said 'magnesium,'" she shares. "And then for a while, he was taking something at midnight, so we had the alarm for that time too."

Support groups were a huge help, a concept Jill believes is integral. During her husband's journey, she periodically cared for him at other health institutions and had a chance to compare. "Mayo Clinic is the only place that created a safe place for caregivers," she says. "And they actually give caregivers equal time." Mayo Clinic's policy states that caregivers must accompany their loved ones to all appointments, which accomplishes two things: It keeps caregivers up to date on their loved ones' needs, and it makes caregivers equal participants in the journey. "It gives caregivers a place. I think that's a really important thing," Jill says.

Support groups also helped Jill understand what to expect. "I found that people sometimes are afraid to bother their medical team with questions." She says caregivers don't want to feel that they're complaining or they're a burden. Having a group to ask a question about what's typical and what's not is extremely helpful.

Taking care of yourself during the transplant journey is another challenge, Jill adds. "Self-care is a hard thing for a caregiver to do," she comments. "Everyone will tell you to take care of yourself, get rest, don't forget to eat and exercise. And the truth is, you really can't do that when you're in crisis mode." Jill recommends doing what you can. Maybe you don't run 5 miles, but you go for a walk. You don't go to a spa, but you take a long bath. Or you simply have quiet time to yourself whenever possible. "Sometimes, in the middle of the night, when Patrick was sleeping, I sat in the dark and looked outside for half an hour and just tried to breathe."

But perhaps the most important thing to remember, Jill notes, is that you're human. That means you'll mess things up every now and then. And when that happens, try not to beat yourself down. "None of us is perfect. We all make mistakes, so forgive yourself for making them," she says. "Give yourself some grace — and keep going."

It's true that you and your loved one just crossed a major milestone. The person in your care has successfully undergone complex surgery and is doing well enough to go home. However, your work isn't over. This is the time when you'll likely need to be with your loved one at all hours, playing several different roles. You'll likely need to be a shopping companion, nurse, cook, chauffeur, note taker and cheerleader.

Similar to when your loved one first left the hospital and was recovering nearby, it's still important that you attend all appointments, take notes, and watch for changes or challenges. And while your loved one may be taking on a bigger role when it comes to medications, it's still important that you provide reminders if necessary and check that the right pills are being taken at the right times. Last but not least, it's up to you to make sure your loved one adheres to all safety guidelines — from food prep to pet interactions — to minimize infection risks.

This is a lot. And wearing so many different hats at once can be exhausting and stressful. But keep in mind that you've already made it this far. And don't be afraid to lean on family members and friends for assistance. Specific requests for help, such as a run to the grocery store or a trip to the pharmacy to pick up a prescription refill, tend to get the best response. Remember that you can't take care of someone else if you don't take care of yourself. Make time in your day for rest and relaxation so that you have energy and strength when needed.

Also keep in mind that although you and your loved one are returning home, that doesn't mean everything will return to "normal." Your loved one may act different from usual at times, including being irritable, aloof, frustrated, sad or forgetful. The person in your care may feel nauseous, have stomachaches or other pains, have difficulty sleeping, or be hungry all the time or not hungry at all. Many of these symptoms are side effects of the antirejection medicines. Pain and exhaustion also can contribute to mood swings or confusion.

Seeing your loved one have these experiences may be difficult. You may be wondering if the changes are permanent and if at some point you'll be able to return to some semblance of normalcy. Chances are many of these difficulties will ease once the person in your care starts taking fewer medications or smaller doses of them. For example, a few months after surgery when your loved one can stop taking steroid medications, side effects such as high blood pressure or diabetes will likely diminish and your loved one may sleep better.

As the person in your care starts feeling stronger and is able to reengage in some favorite pastimes and activities, you'll likely start to develop a more comfortable routine that's better suited to your new normal.

15

Healthy for life

STILL GOING STRONG NEARLY 30 YEARS LATER
PETE'S STORY

If you saw Pete planting crops or feeding his 150 cattle, you'd never guess that the heart beating in his chest isn't the one he was born with. The 64-year-old farmer received a heart transplant in 1997. He's been living with this new heart for nearly 30 years.

Pete was 34 years old when he was diagnosed with cardiomyopathy, a condition that makes it difficult for the heart muscle to pump blood. Pete's heart had become enlarged and no longer functioned effectively. A father of three young children at the time, Pete had been an active, outdoorsy person who played sports in his earlier years before his life took a dramatic, unexpected turn. Pete soon found himself on the transplant waitlist, and he spent 118 days in the hospital with a heart that barely kept beating. It was a difficult time for him, especially being away from his family.

After a couple of chances for a new heart that didn't work out, the news Pete was awaiting finally arrived in late November. "I got my transplant on Thanksgiving Day," Pete says, which gave the holiday a whole new meaning for him. "I have a lot of thanks to give."

Pete says getting used to life after transplant surgery took some time, with the first three months being the hardest. "The transplant itself wasn't so hard, but the antirejection medicines were really tough on a person," Pete shares. "And you didn't know whether you should be out in the public because you were so scared of getting sick because you were on all these medicines." Fortunately, the side effects improved, and life became easier once doctors reduced his medication dosages. "I've tapered down quite a bit. I don't take as much as when I first started," Pete says. "Every year, I do my annual check, and they keep monitoring me."

While some transplant recipients choose to write to their donor families, most don't know their donors, at least not right away. And more often than not, transplant organs come from far away. In Pete's small community, things were different. He received his new heart from a young man who lived 15 miles away and died of injuries due to a bad fall. Pete learned this when the donor family contacted him after his transplant. "His mom called me, like, two months after, because she knew whose heart I got because it was on the news," Pete says. "I was fortunate to meet his family and do things with his family," he adds.

To this day, Pete remains grateful for the donor family's gracious gift of life. Without his new heart, he wouldn't have been able to see his children grow up and get married. Since his transplant, Pete has welcomed 11 grandchildren into the world. He likes telling this story to local high school students every year as part of their driver education instruction as they prepare to take the driver's test. "It's kind of a good story for the kids to see how important transplant is," he says. Pete hopes it will encourage some to consider being organ donors and make this known on their driver's licenses.

Living with a transplanted heart has had its occasional challenges. A few years ago, Pete developed kidney cancer that he thinks may have been a side effect of the antirejection medications, which diminish the immune system's ability to fight tumors. "They said that could happen after so many years," he says. He underwent treatment, beat the cancer and went back to farming. He's had some other, minor issues too. "I think the medicines have kind of started to deteriorate my muscles a little bit, because I'm just not as strong as I used to be," he shares. "I have my aches and pains, but that's because I'm getting to be 65 years old. So I guess that comes with the territory. I think maybe another year or so, once I turn 65, I'll start slowing down a little bit."

Meanwhile, Pete's heart is still going strong nearly 30 years later. He says despite having to take medicines every day and dealing with a few health issues, his life has been pretty typical.

"I'm still really active. I still farm, I still drive a tractor every day and I still have a lot of cattle that I take care of on a daily basis. I plant corn and soybeans, and we put up a lot of hay. I go hunting, I'm active in my church and I go on trips with my wife. I even traveled to Europe — to Germany — because we had an exchange student. So we went there to visit her family for a couple of weeks."

"I'm pretty fortunate," he reflects, "after all these years, to do all that."

After receiving your transplant, and as you begin taking fewer medications and smaller doses over time, you should start feeling better and more energetic. Being back in your own home will probably help too. After a few months, you'll likely be able to do more around the house, including making meals, as well as venture out on your own and start driving again. You'll likely have your medication routine down by this time and know what to refill and when. And because you'll probably need less help from your caregiver, you'll likely feel more independent each day.

You also may find that life is more relaxed without your previous stresses. You no longer have to wait for the transplant call. You don't have to be ready to drop everything and travel to a hospital at a moment's notice.

Having a healthy, working organ also brings more freedom and the ability to do things you couldn't do before. Once your transplant team gives you a go-ahead, you'll likely be able to enjoy long walks or take a vacation.

But your life won't be unrestricted. You'll still need to exercise a lot of caution to minimize your infection risks. It's important to remain vigilant about the food you eat and your interaction with pets. You must avoid people who appear sick. Another important thing to remember is that antirejection medications increase the risk of cancer, especially skin cancer. So protect yourself from the sun's ultraviolet rays when you're outside. The medications also can make you more vulnerable to insect-borne diseases, so it's important to reduce your exposure to ticks and mosquitoes. And if you travel abroad, make sure you have all the right vaccinations for where you're going.

Although many medication side effects will usually decrease once doses are lowered, new issues may develop over time. These may include changes to your hair, nails, skin and gums. While these issues aren't generally dangerous, they may affect your appearance. Nonprescription cosmetics may provide some help. Or you may want to consult a dermatologist or cosmetologist. If you choose to see a specialist, make sure that person knows you received a transplant and is aware of the medications you take. You may need to explain how the medicines work, including your increased risk of infection.

SKIN CARE

Following are skin changes that you may notice over time. Not everyone experiences these changes, and the effects are more bothersome for some people than for others.

Acne

Acne is a common side effect of antirejection medications, specifically the medications sirolimus (Rapamune) and prednisone. Not all transplant recipients develop acne, but many do. The degree of the condition varies.

A nonprescription topical acne treatment may help. If you use cosmetics, purchase makeup that's oil-free and doesn't block pores or promote the formation of blemishes. This type of makeup is often referred to as noncomedogenic.

If these measures don't help, a prescription-strength medication in cream or pill form may work. However, it's recommended that you consult with an experienced dermatology specialist before you take any new medications or use any topical medications. Inform this person of all the medications you take. You don't want your new medication to interact with an existing medication and cause problems. Remember to contact your transplant team before taking any new medication.

Puffy face

Corticosteroid medications, such as prednisone, can cause you to develop a round or puffy face. Makeup may help reduce the appearance of puffiness. Make sure to use oil-free, noncomedogenic makeup.

Spider veins

Spider veins are small, dilated blood vessels near the surface of the skin. Although they may appear anywhere, spider veins typically form on the face and legs. If they appear on your face, they may make it look flushed, as if you have a fever.

Spider veins can be masked with oil-free, noncomedogenic foundation or concealer. They also may be treated with laser therapy. Discuss this option with a dermatologist and your transplant team to determine whether there may be any risks you wouldn't want to take.

Sebaceous hyperplasia

In this condition, little bumps called papules form on the skin due to overly productive oil glands. There's no nonprescription cream, peel or abrasion technique that treats the papules. If you develop them and find them bothersome, talk with a dermatologist about possible self-care steps you can try at home to reduce their development or appearance.

Change in skin color

Some medications can cause a change in the color of your facial skin. The best way to manage a change in skin color is with makeup. Make sure to use an oil-free, noncomedogenic product.

Tanning may seem like an appealing solution to improve your skin color, but it's a dangerous option. Remember that antirejection medicines make you extremely vulnerable to cancer because your immune

SKIN CARE AT A GLANCE

- Examine your skin monthly. Use a mirror or ask a partner to check areas that you can't see. Look for new or changing growths, including patches or spots that have changed color, scaly growths, bleeding areas, or changing moles. Report any changes to your healthcare team.
- Consistently use sunscreen with a sun protection factor (SPF) of 30 or higher on your face, neck, ears, the backs of your hands and the top of your scalp if you have thin hair. Use lip balms that contain sunscreen. Apply sunscreen 30 minutes before going outside and reapply every few hours.
- Wear a broad-brimmed hat, sunglasses and tightly woven, protective clothing when outdoors.
- Avoid the sun during the high-intensity hours between 10 a.m. and 4 p.m.
- Moisturize regularly to maintain your skin's natural moisture level.

system isn't as robust at identifying and destroying cancer cells. Avoid tanning outdoors or by using tanning beds. If you want to look tanned, use a bronzing lotion or spray, sold at drug stores or applied by technicians at beauty salons. It's a safer alternative.

Skin irritation

Your skin may be more sensitive because of the medicines you're taking. Look for skin products that don't contain a lot of chemicals, dyes or perfumes. Keep in mind that hair and nail products also may contain chemicals that can cause skin irritation, such as the chemicals toluene and formaldehyde. Use products that are free of these chemicals.

HAIR CARE

Stressful events, such as severe illness, a high fever, childbirth and major surgery can cause hair loss. Some medications also can increase your risk of hair loss. After transplant surgery, some people start seeing just the opposite: hair in places where it typically doesn't grow.

Hair loss

After your transplant, your hair may thin, and you may develop some bald spots. This may happen six weeks to six months after the surgery and it may continue for up to a year. Your hair will usually regrow again on its own. Medications, particularly antirejection medicines such as tacrolimus (Prograf, Astagraf XL, Envarsus XR), can cause hair to thin.

There are many ways to compensate for thinning hair. They include a new hairstyle, wigs or toupees, scarves, turbans and headbands, and shaving the head. There also are nonprescription products, such as minoxidil (Rogaine, Hair Regrowth for Men, others) that may promote hair regrowth.

Hair loss also may result from a fungal infection of the scalp, called tinea capitis. This type of infection can occur in people whose immune systems are suppressed. The condition is easy to diagnose and is treatable with antifungal medications.

Hair growth

If you're taking the antirejection medication cyclosporine (Sandimmune, Neoral, Gengraf), you may see increased hair growth in areas other than the scalp. You'll likely notice this about 2 to 4 weeks after starting the medication, and it'll continue for as long as you keep taking it. The amount and location of the hair growth varies with each person.

There are several ways of removing the unwanted hair, all of which should be done with caution to avoid breaking or scratching the skin to minimize infection risk. You can use:

- A shaver, razor or tweezers, but be careful to avoid nicking the skin. A cut may let germs enter the body and lead to an infection.
- Topical creams that dissolve hair, but they may irritate the skin.

- Waxing, but keep the wax at a warm, not hot, temperature to avoid burning the skin. Waxing can irritate skin and cause an inflammation of hair follicles and acne breakouts.
- Laser hair removal performed by or supervised by a healthcare professional. This works best for people who have white skin and dark hair.
- Electrolysis, performed by a licensed electrologist. This procedure delivers an electrical current through a needle to destroy the hair root. Because it involves several needle punctures, it increases the chances of infection and thus carries more risks.

NAIL CARE

Transplant recipients can develop dry, brittle nails, and nails that pull away from the nail beds. These issues may result from the illness that led to the organ failure, poor health during organ failure, or stress on the body during and after the transplant surgery.

Visiting a nail salon might seem like a logical solution, but it comes with its own set of issues. Because your immune system is suppressed, you have an increased chance of developing a fungal infection of the nails or a bacterial infection of the cuticles. These infections are hard to treat and often impossible to cure.

If you use a nail salon, buy your own instruments and bring them with you. Make sure to sterilize them after each use by boiling them in water for 20 minutes. Ask salon personnel to avoid pushing, trimming or otherwise manipulating your cuticles. Also, avoid soaking your feet in a tub of water or having someone aggressively scrape your feet because fungal infections can sneak in that way too.

DENTAL CARE

To minimize your risk of infection, avoid nonemergency dental work, including teeth cleanings, during the first six months after transplant surgery. After that, you can resume your regular dental exams and cleanings. If you received a lung or a heart transplant, your transplant team may recommend taking an antibiotic prior to your appointments.

NAIL CARE AT A GLANCE

- Keep your hands, nails and cuticles well moisturized. Use lotion after washing your hands and at bedtime.
- Avoid having professional manicures or pedicures.
- Keep your nails trimmed short, but don't trim the nails so short that you nick the skin beneath the nail.
- Avoid pushing, trimming or otherwise manipulating your cuticles.
- Don't clean beneath the nails with a sharp object or in a rough manner. This may lift the nail off the nail bed and open the skin, raising infection risk.
- File or buff the nails in one direction only. Use a fine-grain buffer and avoid coarse buffers.
- Take 2.5 milligrams of the oral vitamin biotin daily or apply a nail hardener to strengthen your nail plates. Let your health-care team know about any vitamins you take and how much you're taking.
- Use only nonacetone nail polish remover, at most once a week. An acetate remover is best.
- Use toluene-free and formaldehyde-free cosmetics.
- Wear rubber or vinyl gloves if you must keep your hands in water for long periods. If your hands sweat when wearing rubber gloves, wear cotton gloves or liners in them.

Be aware that the medication cyclosporine can cause your gums to thicken and overgrow, a condition called gum hyperplasia. If you develop this condition, good oral hygiene and regular dental visits are especially important to avoid an infection taking hold in your mouth and affecting the rest of your body. If your overgrowth becomes excessive, it may be possible to have the gums trimmed. Speak with your transplant team or your dentist to get a referral to a periodontist, an expert who treats gum disease.

EATING OUT

Dining out is a great pleasure in life. It gives you the opportunity to enjoy foods that you can't or don't have time to prepare yourself — and there's no doing dishes afterward! Plus, dining out is a great way to socialize and spend time with friends and family or to celebrate special occasions. Be careful, however, when dining out, and remember food safety precautions.

When eating away from home, ordering an item from a menu is generally safer than eating from a buffet or taking part in a potluck. With a buffet or potluck, serving utensils are touched by multiple people, and the utensils can easily become contaminated with germs. From there, the germs can transfer onto your hands and onto the food itself. Food at a buffet or potluck also may become contaminated if someone who is sick coughs or sneezes when going through the food line.

When selecting a restaurant, pay attention to its cleanliness. Also, order foods that you believe are safe. Your food at a restaurant should be cooked as thoroughly as it is at home. This means that foods such as sushi, sashimi or ceviche aren't safe options. If you're ordering a salad, you may want to ask how the greens and lettuces are cleaned and whether the dressings have any raw egg ingredients in them. When choosing drinks and desserts, make sure they don't contain grapefruit, Seville oranges, pomegranates or pomelos, which can interfere with your antirejection medications.

Finally, avoid dishes with bean sprouts and alfalfa sprouts. These greens are grown in warm and humid conditions that are good not only for sprout germination but also bacterial growth. These foods can harbor *Escherichia (E.) coli,* salmonella and listeria, among other pathogens. Even when thoroughly washed, they may still contain trace amounts of bacteria.

OUTDOOR ACTIVITIES

As you begin to feel better, you'll likely want to do many things that you may not have been able to enjoy in a while. This may involve spending time outside.

- Make sure that the restaurant or cafe you choose has a high food hygiene rating, which is usually displayed on the premises.
- Avoid high-risk foods such as uncooked or raw meat and seafood.
- Avoid raw or undercooked eggs in sauces, desserts and dressings such as homemade mayonnaise, homemade ice cream, chocolate mousse, meringue, and hollandaise and bearnaise sauces. If you're not sure, ask the chef how the food is prepared.
- If ordering salads or a dish with raw vegetables, ask how the produce is cleaned.
- Ask about the ingredients in juices, iced teas, desserts and preserves to ensure they don't contain grapefruits, Seville oranges, pomegranates, pomelos or any other ingredients that can interfere with your antirejection medications.
- Choose dishes that are cooked to order and that arrive hot and thoroughly cooked.
- Avoid rice that's precooked and kept warm, which is often done in Chinese and Indian restaurants. Ask for freshly cooked rice or select something else.
- Avoid buffets due to the risk that the food may be contaminated by other diners, particularly if it's a self-service buffet at which the same serving spoons are used by many people.

Sun care

Antirejection medications make you more vulnerable to cancer because your immune system is less robust at finding and destroying cancer cells. This is particularly true for skin cancer. That's why when you're outside, make sure to protect yourself from getting sunburned. Use sunscreen with an SPF of 30 or higher and reapply it often. Wear a hat and protective clothing, especially if you'll be outside for a long time. If you notice any skin changes, make an appointment with a dermatologist.

Swimming or bathing

Swimming and bathing are great forms of exercise and recreation, but not all bodies of water are safe, especially if you've had a transplant. Swimming or bathing in fresh water has a higher risk of infection; therefore, it's best not to swim or bathe in ponds, lakes, creeks, rivers or streams.

Swimming or bathing in chlorinated pools or the ocean is generally considered safe. It's best, however, to avoid hot tubs, jacuzzis and steam rooms because bacteria tend to breed in hot and humid environments. Additionally, if you have any open sores or cuts on your skin, don't swim or bathe until they heal.

Insect-borne diseases

Insect-borne diseases are spread by mosquitoes and ticks. They include West Nile virus infection, Lyme disease and Rocky Mountain spotted fever, among others. Such diseases can cause severe illness if you've had a transplant.

To protect yourself from tick and mosquito bites, wear long-sleeved shirts and long pants, avoid being around stagnant water, and make sure windows and doors have screens on them. After walking in grassy or wooded areas, inspect yourself for ticks. And use insect repellents that contain one of the following ingredients:

- DEET.
- Picaridin.
- IR3535.
- Oil of lemon eucalyptus.
- Para-menthane-diol.
- 2-Undecanone.

EXERCISE

About eight weeks after your transplant surgery, if you're doing well, your transplant team will likely encourage you to begin exercising.

Start with moderate exercise. The form of exercise you engage in will likely depend on your preferences and on the type of transplant you received.

Unless you're told otherwise, you should be able to engage in most sports and activities, but you'll likely be told to avoid heavy contact sports such as boxing, martial arts or football. With these activities, there's a risk of damage to your new organ.

Activities you might consider include walking, jogging, biking, playing golf or tennis, swimming in a chlorinated pool, taking a yoga or Pilates class, and dancing. If you're not sure if the form of exercise you prefer is safe, talk with your transplant team.

As time goes on, try to make exercise and physical activity a regular part of your daily routine. This can help improve your health, fitness and stamina. Exercise and physical activity also can help you manage your weight, strengthen your bones, increase your energy level, and feel less anxious or stressed.

TOBACCO AND ALCOHOL USE

Avoid tobacco use in any form — smoking or chewing — after transplant surgery. Studies show that using tobacco can negatively affect the healing process, reducing the success of transplanted tissues being accepted by the body. Tobacco also can aggravate the side effects of medications taken after transplant surgery.

Nicotine found in tobacco products also can cause vasospasm, which is a narrowing of the blood vessels. This can lead to blood clots in the arteries to your new organ. Blood clots can cause the new organ to fail.

Also avoid electronic cigarettes, commonly referred to as vaping devices or e-cigarettes. The liquid used in e-cigarettes contains nicotine.

Whether you can drink alcohol depends on several factors including the type of transplant you received, the medications you're taking and your personal health history. The best advice is to not drink alcohol until discussing it with your transplant team.

CANNABIS

Many states and the District of Columbia have introduced medical cannabis programs, but products containing cannabis pose certain risks for transplant recipients. The terms *cannabis* and *marijuana* are often used synonymously. Marijuana is made from parts of the cannabis plant that contain the compound delta-9-tetrahydrocannabinol (THC).

Smoking marijuana can increase the risk of lung fungal infections. If you choose to smoke marijuana, either bake it in the oven at 300 degrees Fahrenheit for 15 minutes or microwave it for at least 10 seconds to kill fungal spores. Baking marijuana before eating it — such as by adding it to brownies or cakes — also will reduce fungal infection risk.

There are other concerns. Whether smoked or ingested, it's possible that some marijuana components may alter the levels of your antirejection medications. Unfortunately, it's not yet known to what extent marijuana can interfere with these medications. Cannabis is composed of two major compounds, THC and cannabidiol (CBD). Research suggests that products that contain only THC may be safer to use. However, more research is needed on all products that contain THC or CBD to better determine their health risks and potential interactions.

TRAVEL

If your recovery goes well, you'll be able to travel six months to a year after your transplant — as long as you follow the recommended health guidelines. If you're traveling to other countries, you may need to exercise extra caution.

For example, in some countries you should avoid drinking or even brushing your teeth with tap water. You might consider packing a small kettle so you can boil water to drink or to wash fruits and vegetables if bottled water isn't available. Don't drink beverages containing ice cubes, as the ice cubes may come from tap water. It's also a good idea not to eat food from street vendors, as they may use ice cubes to keep their food ingredients cool.

Research your trip before going. Are there any infectious diseases prevalent at your destination? Are they less or more common during certain seasons? Will you need specific vaccines or booster shots for diseases such as tetanus or hepatitis?

If you need to get vaccinated, avoid receiving live vaccines. Some vaccines need several weeks to work, so make your appointment at least a month before your trip. Make sure to research what type of healthcare is available at your destination and whether your health insurance will cover you. Additionally, you may consider buying medical evacuation insurance.

Avoid petting or touching local animals on your trip. Use sunscreen and insect repellent. Wash your hands with soap regularly and use hand sanitizer. If you're traveling to a place where malaria is

CONTACTING THE DONOR FAMILY

As you begin to feel better, you may start thinking more about the person whose organ you received. Grateful for the gift of life that you've been given, you may want to thank the donor's family personally.

There's a way to do it. Organ procurement organizations can facilitate conversations between transplant recipients and donor families. You can write the donor's family a letter or send a card of thanks. Different transplant hospitals have different procedures for contacting donor families. Ask your transplant social worker where to mail your card or letter, as it may differ depending on what organ procurement organization was involved.

To begin, find a card or some stationery that's beautiful and peaceful. And write on it when you're in a positive mood. Acknowledge your deepest sympathy for the loss of the family's loved one and offer your sincere thanks and gratitude for your new chance at life as a result of their gift. Many donor families appreciate such messages.

In your letter or card, you might include a bit of information about yourself and your family. You also can tell the donor's family prevalent, you'll need protection against it. Some malaria medications may interfere with your antirejection medicines, so discuss this with your transplant team.

When packing your medications, bring extras in case of unexpected travel delays. If you'll be changing time zones, talk with a pharmacist or your healthcare team for help in adjusting your medication schedule. Always place your medications in your carry-on bag and have them in their original bottles in case questions from airport security staff arise. Finally, avoid people who appear sick and consider wearing a mask on airplanes, trains, subways and buses.

what you've been able to do since you received your transplant — for example, going back to school, getting married, watching your children graduate college or watching your grandchildren grow. Also, describe the type of donation you received. Some donors contribute multiple organs, and they often go to different people.

It's important to remain anonymous and not give too much information identifying yourself, such as your age, your name, where you live or where you work. It's also best not to include information regarding the medical center where you received your transplant or your surgeon's name. And it's generally best to avoid any religious messages or information regarding your religious affiliation out of respect to the donor family's faith tradition.

It's impossible to know whether the donor family will write back. Families have their own ways of dealing with grief and loss. Some donor families choose to stay private and won't write back. Others find that corresponding about their loved one helps them in their grieving process. In some cases, if both you and the donor family are willing, the organ procurement organization can organize a meeting, and you can share your gratitude in person.

INTIMACY

Sexuality is part of being human. Love, affection and intimacy all play a role in healthy relationships. You can resume intimacy and sexual activity when you're comfortable, but it's advisable to wait until your incision fully heals, which generally occurs about 6 to 8 weeks after surgery. To avoid straining the incision site or your recovering body, you may want to use a low-stress position. If you have any pain, it's best to adjust the position.

Transplant surgery and the medications you're taking may change the way you view your body. They also may affect your ability to be intimate with your partner. For example, male transplant recipients may experience challenges with erections after surgery. This might be due to reduced blood flow to the penis or be a consequence of the transplant medicines. Usually, these challenges can be managed with medications, but it's possible you may have to find new ways to be intimate and express your love. Before you take medications to treat erectile dysfunction, discuss their use with your transplant team. It's also important to be open with your partner about your feelings, concerns and needs and speak with your transplant team about any concerns you have.

PREGNANCY

Having a child can be a wonderful experience. However, for individuals who've received an organ transplant, pregnancy comes with high risk. Some antirejection medications, particularly the drugs mycophenolate mofetil (CellCept, Myhibbin) and mycophenolic sodium (Myfortic), increase the risk of birth defects. The medications also can increase the risk of miscarriage.

If you're taking these medications and would like to have a child, let your transplant team know. This applies to people of all genders. Your transplant team will likely want to replace the medicine with a different type of antirejection medication to reduce the risk of birth defects and pregnancy loss.

There are other risks too. Pregnancy can increase your risk of organ rejection. The seriousness of the risk depends in part on your and your partner's human leukocyte antigens, commonly referred to as HLAs. (You can read more about HLAs on pages 35-36.) If your partner's HLAs are similar to your donor's HLAs, your body will contain an increased amount of these HLAs as your baby develops. This usually isn't a problem during pregnancy itself because the placenta separates your baby's blood circulation from your own. But it may become life-threatening as you give birth.

During the birthing process, tissues and fluids intermix, and the influx of HLAs can cause your body to ramp up its antibody production. A sudden increase in antibodies can overpower your antirejection medications, allowing the antibodies to attack your new organ and damage or destroy it.

If you're thinking about becoming pregnant, discuss this with your transplant team so that you fully understand the risks to both you and your baby. If you choose to pursue pregnancy, your transplant team may want to adjust your medications to increase the chances of a safer pregnancy with less risk to your baby. If you determine that you don't want to become pregnant, make sure to use birth control and discuss your options with the team. Even if your periods seem to have stopped, you should always use birth control after a transplant.

FOR CAREGIVERS: STEPPING BACK

Watching your loved one recover and become more self-reliant may be the most rewarding part of being a caregiver. As the weeks go by, you'll likely see that the person in your care is growing stronger and becoming more independent. As your loved one's health improves and more activity is possible, you may see the person going out, taking walks, exercising, returning to work and enjoying activities that weren't possible while waiting for the transplant.

That means that you've done your job well. You've taken your loved one through a grueling and challenging journey. You were there 24/7 for weeks and months, and you've gotten through the most difficult parts. Now you can take a breather and watch as your loved one improves with every passing day.

There will probably still be some things that your loved one may need help with. For example, it's still best that your loved one not clean cat litter boxes if you have them. When it's time for a checkup at the transplant center, the person in your care may want a travel companion. The individual also may need your help with occasional tasks and appointments. But overall, you can take a step back and attend to things you haven't been able to do while you were a full-time caregiver.

Reaching this mark on your caregiving journey may leave you feeling both exhilarated and exhausted. You also may feel anxious about your loved one's future. Or you may feel traumatized by experiences you've recently been through. These feelings are fairly common.

Research finds that approximately 7% of transplant caregivers experience anxiety, about 25% have post-traumatic stress disorder, and about a third deal with depression and so-called adjustment disorder, a heightened reaction to stress that involves negative thoughts and strong emotions.

If that's how you're feeling, it's time to take care of yourself. Try focusing on things you enjoy doing. Stay in touch with your caregiver support groups. Make time to visit family and friends. Enjoy a spa visit. Consider taking meditation or yoga classes to relieve stress and boost your moods. Or let someone take care of you now and then. You've been through a grueling experience from which you also may need to recover. You, too, deserve a little bit of "me time!"

16

At home with your child

As parents, you've already faced the uncertainty that comes with your child's health challenges. Now you're stepping into new territory — caring for your child after transplant surgery. It's natural to feel anxious about what lies ahead — how to manage the medications, prevent infections and ensure that your child's recovery is as smooth as possible.

Ongoing medical care, including regular healthcare visits and testing, is required for the rest of your child's life to monitor your child's overall health and the health of the transplanted organ.

The initial period following surgery is marked by close monitoring and care. If you don't live near your child's transplant hospital, you'll be asked to stay close by. This immediate recovery period — when the odds of organ rejection are highest and medications will need to be adjusted — lasts several weeks. These frequent follow-up visits are crucial for monitoring your child's progress.

If your child is doing well after the initial recovery period, you can return home. This chapter focuses on the period after you return home. You'll still need to follow a regular schedule for checkup visits, but the visits won't be as frequent. Though your child's checkups may not happen as often, they remain extremely important to help catch early signs of rejection or infection. Checkups also are a good time to ask questions about any transplant-related issues your child may be facing.

CHECKUPS: WHAT TO EXPECT

Follow-up visits with the transplant team are critical to ensure that your child's new organ is functioning well and the systems within the body are adjusting to medications. Appointments with the transplant care team will be fairly frequent after your child first returns home, typically every month or so. Over time, the visits will taper down to about once or twice a year. However, your child may need to have lab tests more frequently at your local clinic or hospital. The results of these tests are sent to your transplant team.

A checkup with the transplant team may include routine blood work, urine tests, biopsies, imaging and other diagnostic tests. For example, testing can measure the level of waste products in the blood and help the transplant care team evaluate your child's kidney or liver health. Lab tests also determine the levels of transplant medications in the body. Elevated medication levels can suppress the immune system too much and significantly increase the risk of infection. Meanwhile, levels that are too low don't offer enough protection from rejection. Having low levels of antirejection medicine in the body can lead to a transplant rejection episode.

Routine testing is where potential issues with an organ are often first flagged. That's why it's important for your child to attend all regularly scheduled visits.

Many children are at risk of high blood pressure because of their transplant medications, so you'll need to take your child's blood pressure at home and keep a log to show the team during visits.

If your child has had a kidney transplant, it's vital to track urine output. Any significant decrease in the amount of urine, changes in urine color or the presence of blood should be reported immediately, as these can indicate an issue with the organ.

Sometimes there are delays in growth and development. Delays may depend on how sick your child was before the transplant, as well as the length of time for recovery. Talk to the transplant team about what to expect.

Once you return home, work with your child's primary healthcare professional to monitor your child's growth and development during the months and years after transplant surgery. Try not to compare your child's growth to that of other children. If you have any questions or concerns, be sure to bring them up with your child's healthcare team.

MANAGING MEDICATIONS

A key part of care after transplant surgery is your child's medication regimen. Antirejection medications, also known as immunosuppressants, are medicines that your child will take for life. They can be grouped into two phases:

- **After transplant.** Right after transplant surgery, your child will receive several antirejection medications, often at high doses. This is when the risk of rejection is highest.
- **Maintenance.** After a few months, often doses of the medications are gradually reduced to minimize side effects. Some medicines may be stopped.

It's important that you and your child know the names of each medicine, what the medicine is for, and when and how to take it. You also need to know what to do if your child accidentally misses a dose.

Before leaving the hospital, the transplant team will create a medication plan. At each visit, you'll review and possibly update the plan. It's important to follow this plan exactly, while keeping in mind that medicines and dosages may change frequently based on your child's health.

Your child may need other medicines in addition to antirejection medications. For example, some heart transplant recipients may take medicine to stabilize the heart rhythm. Transplant recipients also may take a supplement to keep electrolyte levels stable.

Make sure that your child receives the medications at the same time and in the same way. For example, some medicines should be taken with food. Setting an alarm or using a smartphone or an app as a reminder can help ensure the medicines are taken on time. Pill organizers also are a good way to help avoid missed or double doses.

Other things to consider:

- Don't stop a medicine or change how much you give unless your child's transplant team tells you to do so. If your child is experiencing side effects, contact the transplant care team immediately.
- Some medicines, such as antibiotics, may interfere with antirejection medications. If your child's primary healthcare professional prescribes a new medication, make sure to contact your child's transplant team. Be aware that nonprescription medicines, supplements and certain foods can interfere with some antirejection medicines. Always talk to your child's transplant team before giving your child anything that's not a part of the regular regimen.
- Bring a list of your child's medicines and doses when you see another medical professional or when you go to a pharmacy.
- Ask the transplant care team what to do if your child misses a dose or if your child vomits after taking the medicine.
- For consistency, try to get the same brand of medicine from the same manufacturer each time the medicine is refilled.
- Mark on a calendar when you need to pick up refills so that you don't run out.

INFECTION PREVENTION

Antirejection medications help your child's immune system fight off germs. Some of the most common infections a child may have after an organ transplant include the following:

COVID-19

Transplant recipients face a higher risk of hospitalization if they develop coronavirus disease 2019 (COVID-19). Ideally, transplant recipients should receive COVID-19 vaccinations before transplant for the best antibody response. Self-care steps to control infections can reduce the risk of a COVID-19 infection.

Cytomegalovirus

Cytomegalovirus (CMV) infection may occur early in life. Afterward, the virus lies dormant, also known as inactive, in the body. Years later, it can wake up, also known as reactivate, and lead to another infection. If your child hasn't been exposed to the virus before the transplant, an infection can occur from the new organ if the donor had CMV. Or your child may develop CMV from exposure after transplant surgery. A blood test for the virus can show the transplant team whether your child is at risk of the infection. An antiviral medicine given after the transplant can help prevent CMV.

Epstein-Barr virus

Epstein-Barr virus (EBV) causes infectious mononucleosis. Mononucleosis also is known as mono. The infection can be severe in children who've received transplants.

Epstein-Barr virus, similar to CMV, becomes dormant in the body. If your child wasn't infected with EBV before the transplant, it can spread from the new organ if the donor had it. A child who hasn't had EBV is at greater risk of the virus after transplant surgery because of a weakened immune system. EBV can lead to post-transplant lymphoproliferative disease (PTLD). This is a type of immune system cancer.

NUTRITION

Good nutrition plays a key role in healing and recovery after a transplant. Depending on the type of transplant your child receives, the transplant care team may provide specific dietary guidelines. Recommendations may include the following:

- Eat foods that provide vitamin D and calcium, such as low-fat milk, cheese and yogurt. Vitamin D and calcium can help reduce the risk of bone weakening due to long-term use of the steroid prednisone. A vitamin D supplement also may be prescribed.
- Follow a heart-healthy diet to lower the risk of high cholesterol, which can be caused by some transplant medications. This includes limiting saturated fats found in red meats and oils, such as palm and coconut oils, and increasing fiber intake by eating foods such as fruits, vegetables and whole-grain products. If your child is

on a low-sodium diet, don't add salt to your child's foods. When you cook, use salt sparingly, if at all. Limit or avoid foods that are processed and high in salt, such as fast foods or sandwich meats. Choose fresh, unprocessed foods as much as you can.

- Avoid simple sugars found in sweets and some sodas and juices, and limit snacking. This can help reduce weight gain caused by some medications.
- Handle food safely. Because your child's immune system is immunocompromised, it's crucial to avoid foodborne infections. Use

REDUCING INFECTION RISK

Following are steps to help minimize the risk of infections. See Chapter 14 for more on infection control strategies.

- **Hand-washing.** Make sure everyone in your household washes their hands frequently with soap and water, especially before eating, after using the restroom and after outdoor activities. Place alcohol-based hand sanitizers around the house for easy access.
- **Exposure.** For the first few months after a transplant, it's important to avoid or limit places where your child might be exposed to germs, such as malls, theaters and child care centers. People who are sick generally shouldn't have contact with your child.
- **Vaccinations.** Make sure your child and your family receive all recommended vaccines. Family members need to be fully vaccinated, especially for the flu and COVID-19, to help protect your child. Most live vaccines — including measles, mumps, rubella (MMR), chickenpox, also called varicella, and the flu nasal mist — aren't appropriate for your child due to the risk of infection from the vaccine itself. The weakened virus or bacteria in a live vaccine potentially can replicate and cause illness in the body of someone on antirejection medications with a compromised immune system. Ask your transplant care team which form of vaccine is recommended for your family. Typically, children may

separate cutting boards for raw meats and other foods. Avoid raw or undercooked meat or seafood. And ensure that leftovers are stored properly.

- Encourage your child to drink plenty of water, unless otherwise advised by your child's transplant team. Dehydration can affect the function of the transplanted organ. Water from your home faucet is considered safe if it comes from a city water supply. It also is considered safe if it comes from a municipal well that serves a highly populated area. Well water from private or small

start receiving vaccines again several months after the transplant. Your child's transplant care team may recommend a different schedule or doses for vaccines than what is typical.

- **Food safety.** Ensure proper food hygiene by cooking meats thoroughly and washing fruits and vegetables.
- **Pets.** Avoid scratches and bites from pets. Don't have your child clean litter boxes or come in contact with any other pet waste. Don't keep birds, rodents, amphibians or reptiles as pets.
- **Dental care.** Regular dental visits are important for children taking antirejection medications to prevent a relatively minor problem from quickly becoming a major one, such as an abscess. Some medicines also may trigger gum disease. However, you'll want to ask your child's transplant care team when to resume dental visits. Some transplant centers recommend waiting at least three months after a transplant and prescribe use of antibiotics before any dental visits.

Be on the lookout for signs of an infection, which include fever or chills, cough or shortness of breath, sore throat or mouth sores, urinary symptoms such as burning or frequent urination, and swelling pain or a change in skin color at the surgical site.

community wells isn't considered safe until you have it tested and approved.

Weight gain or loss may indicate issues with organ function. Weigh your child regularly and report significant changes to the transplant care team.

EXERCISE AND SPORTS

Physical activity, when recommended by the transplant team, can support your child's recovery and general well-being. It also can help counteract some of the side effects of transplant medications, such as heart disease, weight gain, high blood pressure and diabetes. Participating in sports and other physical activities also provides important social interaction. And it helps decrease anxiety and depression.

Aim for 60 minutes of physical activity each day for your child. After surgery, your child likely will need to limit certain activities while the incision is healing. Depending on the organ that's transplanted, limitations may include:

- Lifting anything heavy. The transplant team can offer guidance on this. Generally, avoid lifting anything that is 10 pounds — about the weight of a gallon of milk — or heavier for at least eight weeks after surgery.
- Any activities that require pushing or pulling. Avoid these activities for the first two months after a transplant.
- Rough play. Avoid this for the first two months after surgery.
- Contact sports or any activity that could result in a blow to the transplanted organ. Avoid this for the first three months after a transplant.

Walking is one of the best exercises after transplant surgery. Swimming in a chlorinated pool or the ocean is another option, provided the incision has healed and there are no open cuts or wounds. Freshwater ponds, lakes and other bodies of water are more likely to contain potentially infectious microorganisms.

Check with the transplant team before getting started on other activities, especially participation in sports or other strenuous activities.

BACK TO SCHOOL

One of the most significant transitions after transplant surgery is the return to school. Seeing friends again and engaging in the daily routines of childhood can be a relief for children. However, your child may face some challenges, especially if your child has missed a lot of school or feels different from peers because of the medical condition.

Your child's transplant team will work with you to determine when it's safe for your child to return to school and participate in extracurricular activities. Work with school staff to develop an individualized education plan (IEP) or 504 plan that accommodates your child's medical needs, such as medication schedules, rest periods and infection control measures. Certain safeguards may be necessary, such as implementing dietary steps to avoid foodborne infections or taking precautions to avoid kids who are sick. Inform the school of your child's increased risk of infection so appropriate measures can be taken to ensure your child's safety.

The timing of your child's return to school depends on the length of recovery and individual health. A gradual return may be advised. Accommodations such as shortened school days or extra breaks may be needed.

Teachers, school counselors and friends can play a vital role in helping your child feel included and supported during this transition. Educating teachers and classmates about the transplant and your child's ongoing medical needs can foster understanding and reduce the feeling of isolation.

Work with school staff to make sure your child's peers are educated about organ transplant in an age-appropriate way. This can help prevent teasing or misunderstandings. Encourage school staff to create an inclusive and supportive environment.

WHEN COMPLICATIONS ARISE

Even with careful management, complications such as infection, medication side effects or organ rejection can arise. Early detection is key to addressing these issues before they escalate.

Medication side effects

The antirejection medications your child takes each day can produce various side effects, such as increased appetite, mood swings or increased body hair. Long-term use also may lead to more serious complications, including increased risk of infection, kidney damage, bone loss, high blood pressure, high cholesterol and diabetes.

Some of these side effects may be treated with more medications to help manage them. Other medications that your child takes may include the following:

- Blood pressure medication to lower blood pressure.
- Insulin injections or other diabetes medications to treat high blood sugar.
- Antifungal medicines, also called antifungals, to prevent fungal infections of the mouth, lungs, digestive track, skin and other parts of the body. Because antifungals can affect the levels of anti-rejection medicines, adjustments may be needed to your child's antirejection medicine regimen.
- Antibiotic medicines to treat or prevent bacterial infections.
- Antiviral medicines to treat or prevent infections in the herpes virus family, including CMV, EBV, herpes zoster, which causes chickenpox and shingles, and herpes simplex, which causes cold sores.

Because of the antirejection medicines they take, children who've had transplants also face a higher risk of certain types of cancer. These include skin cancer, a type of lymphoma called post-transplant lympho-proliferative disorder (PTLD), and certain genital warts that can cause cancer.

- Make sure your child takes precautions to be protected from the sun, including using sunscreen with an SPF of 30 or higher regularly. Other precautions include avoiding peak sunlight between 10 a.m. and 2 p.m. and covering up skin as much as possible when outside. Your child also needs to have regular skin checks.
- PTLD risk is greatest in the first year after transplant. It is marked by uncontrolled growth of white blood cells. Treatment may involve reducing antirejection medicines and possibly chemotherapy.

- Taking antirejection medicines makes it harder for the body to fight off human papillomavirus (HPV), which may lead to an increased number of larger warts. If warts are a problem, schedule a visit with a dermatologist or another professional who is experienced with warts. Genital warts can cause cancer in the future, so the HPV vaccine is recommended for both boys and girls. The vaccine is available to those as young as 9 years old.

Growth issues

Children and adolescents who receive a liver transplant may have shorter heights than do other children. Among those who receive a liver transplant, around 75% are below average height five years after the surgery. More than half of young kidney transplant recipients don't reach their expected final height.

This type of side effect isn't always preventable. But research indicates that a shorter duration of steroid medicines along with having transplant surgery at a younger age and maintaining good organ function are related to attaining a more typical height.

Eating a healthy diet and following guidance from a dietitian about recommended calorie levels and vitamin supplementation may help a child reach maximum growth.

Cognitive development

More than one-third of childhood organ transplant recipients have learning disabilities as a result of chronic disease and immune system suppression. Experts recommend screening for children and referral to state-based early intervention programs if they're under age 3. Older children can seek services through their schools and may receive certain educational accommodations.

Organ rejection

This is one of the primary concerns after transplant. Though it's a scary word, *rejection* doesn't mean a transplant is lost. Rather, your child's immune system views the new organ as tissue that "doesn't belong" and it begins to mount a response against the organ.

Episodes of rejection are common. They may happen rather suddenly, occurring within the first few months after a transplant. Or

WHAT IS TRANSPLANT LOSS?

Organ re-transplantation is the process of removing a transplanted organ that no longer works properly and replacing it with a new organ. This can occur because of:

- Chronic rejection.
- Infection.
- Surgical complications.
- Disease recurrence.
- Not following a treatment regimen.
- A transplanted organ that's reached its maximum lifespan.

Transplant loss is not rare. About 25% of children and adolescents on pediatric kidney transplant waitlists have already had one transplant. Re-transplantation in children poses some unique risks.

- **Increased immune response.** Re-transplantation poses a higher risk of rejection because, based on the previous transplant, a child's immune system is more likely to view the new organ as tissue that doesn't belong.
- **Surgical complications.** Similar to any major surgery, there's a risk of bleeding, infection and injury to surrounding tissues. Prior transplant surgery also can make re-transplantation more difficult for a surgeon from a procedural standpoint.
- **Lower success rates.** Some re-transplantation surgeries, such as heart re-transplants, are typically less successful than other types. Success rates for repeat liver and kidney transplants vary. Some studies show success rates similar to the original transplants, and other studies show poorer outcomes.

If your child experiences transplant loss, the transplant team will advise how to best move forward. Going back on a waitlist may be advised to offer your child the best chance of recovery and typical childhood development.

they can happen later. Early rejections, often called acute rejections, are generally the most treatable.

Rejections that occur later over a longer period of time are known as chronic rejections. A chronic rejection can gradually reduce organ function. This can be hard to treat and may eventually lead to organ failure. Chronic rejection is one of the most common reasons for transplant loss.

Rejection is most easily recognized and treated in liver and kidney transplants through routine blood tests that monitor organ function. Routine ultrasound scans are used to monitor heart transplants. Some newer blood tests to help check for rejection also are being developed.

Usually, signs or symptoms aren't present yet when rejection is detected early. Signs and symptoms such as fever, pain, changes in organ function, jaundice and swelling are indications that the body is starting to reject a transplanted organ. A biopsy of the organ is often necessary to confirm that rejection is the cause of a change in organ function.

To treat rejection, the transplant care team typically will adjust the dosages of the antirejection medications your child takes. The care team may prescribe more medications. These medicines may need to be administered intravenously by way of an IV. Sometimes this may require a hospital stay. Early detection and prompt treatment are crucial to preventing irreversible damage.

EMOTIONAL IMPACTS

Emotional and psychological recovery after a pediatric transplant can be as significant as the physical healing. Children may experience a range of emotions following the procedure — relief, fear, anxiety or even confusion about what happened to them. Depending on their age, they may not fully understand the surgery or the long-term requirements for staying healthy.

For younger children, the trauma of surgery and frequent medical visits can cause anxiety or fear of future procedures. Adolescents, meanwhile, may struggle with the reality of daily medications, having to take added health precautions and feeling different from their peers.

Parents and caregivers also face their own emotional challenges, ranging from relief and gratitude to ongoing anxiety about the future health of the child in their care. The period before transplant surgery may have been filled with stress and fear. Adjusting to the changes after surgery also takes time for everyone.

Psychological support from therapists and counselors who specialize in pediatric care, as well as from transplant-specific support groups, can be invaluable. Your child's transplant team can set you up with the necessary resources to address your and your child's mental health needs.

Family dynamics
The impact of a pediatric transplant affects the entire family. Parents often find themselves balancing the needs of their recovering child with the needs of siblings, work responsibilities and their own emotional well-being. The demands of caregiving, particularly in the early stages after a transplant, can be overwhelming. Siblings may feel neglected or jealous of all the attention a brother or sister is receiving. Or they may worry about their sibling's health.

Open communication within the family is essential for maintaining strong relationships and ensuring that everyone's needs are met. Support networks, including extended family, friends and transplant support groups, can be valuable resources for families.

Connecting with others who've been through similar experiences can provide both practical advice and emotional support in a journey that can often be overwhelming. Keep in mind that with patience, resilience and your guidance, your child will be well on the way to healing and better days ahead.

17

Through adolescence and beyond

LETTING A TEEN BE A TEEN
BRAXTON AND MELISSA'S STORY

"We don't put hearts in kids so that they have to live in a bubble. We put hearts in kids so that they can live."

Melissa carries with her these words from one of her son's doctors. As she and her family navigate life after her son's emergency heart transplant, the power of this sentiment helps her keep perspective and lets her son be as typical a teen as possible.

Her son, Braxton, had just turned 16 in early 2024 when an infection with the childhood virus parvovirus B19 — more commonly referred to as fifth disease — caused his immune system to attack and break down his heart muscle. It's a rare complication that left his heart having trouble beating. A transplant was his only option for survival.

Fortunately, a donor heart was found within a week and the transplant was a success, but there were complications. Among them was compartment syndrome, a muscle and nerve condition triggered by the virus that required emergency surgery to remove some of Braxton's leg muscles.

"I'll be honest: Braxton's complications were mentally exhausting and all-consuming," Melissa says. "There were so many of them and they just kept coming." She recalls panicking at the smallest setbacks, and her worry began to leave her with unending negative thoughts. Meeting with a therapist helped her learn to change how she was processing those thoughts, she says.

Members of Braxton's medical team also offered assurance. "They told me that it will be an uphill battle with steps forward and stumbles backward, but as long as the trajectory was forward, we were on the right path," she says. With this guidance, she concentrated on each complication and how to manage it that day — leaving the future to, well, the future.

Still, Melissa can't help thinking ahead. She still fears for Braxton's health and wonders how long his transplant will last. But she also recognizes that some things are beyond anyone's control. "I learned from Braxton, who'd say, 'Mom, stop worrying about the things you can't control and focus your energy and thoughts on what you can control.'"

Like following the antirejection protocol. Braxton carefully adheres to the rigorous routine required to ensure his body doesn't reject the new heart. He knows the names of the medications he takes, their dosage, and which ones are taken when, either at 8 a.m. or 8 p.m. He remembers to bring them with him if he's not going to be home at those times. Because of complications from the virus, he also regularly meets with specialists in a range of disciplines, including physical therapy, nephrology and infectious disease, in addition to his transplant team.

Braxton's diligence in following his treatment plan has made it easier for Melissa to let her child live his life. Braxton is slowly getting back into the sports he enjoyed before he got sick, such as wrestling. "There are many things that Braxton wanted to do and still wants to do that make me a little uneasy," she says. "There are immunosuppression restrictions. But I'm still able to let him be a teenager."

A recent hunting trip in Wyoming — complete with camping in the mountains and limited cell service — put it all in perspective. "I'd rather have him be out there living life and enjoying his passions than sitting at home, unhappy being 'safe,'" she says.

Melissa understands how all this can seem overwhelming at first, and the thought of letting your child be active again is daunting. "It's a long road, a marathon really," she says. "The beginning of this journey is tough — emotionally and physically — but it gets better. You adjust. What seems overwhelming eventually becomes a normal way of life later. Is your life different? Yes. Does that make it bad? No! There is life after a heart transplant. And it's a full life."

Your child's adolescent years are a time of rapid physical, emotional and social development. Guiding teens through this phase is challenging enough. But when your child also is an organ transplant recipient, the stakes can feel higher. Understandably so, in some ways.

Adolescence marks a high-risk period for transplant failure. There are likely multiple reasons for this. Teens are exploring their independence and testing boundaries, making some of them more likely to engage in risk-taking behavior and less likely to follow treatment plans. Sometimes, unintentional behavior — such as simple forgetfulness — is to blame.

The teen years also are a time when healthcare is starting to transition from pediatrics to adult care. This shift can be overwhelming as teens move from their familiar pediatric transplant care, with teams that have a more hands-on approach, to adult transplant care with new team members and additional responsibilities. Add to this a robust immune system that's more likely to respond to a transplanted organ, causing rejection and organ failure risks to rise. Researchers continue to look for ways to reduce rejection and organ failure in adolescents.

As a parent, however, it's critical to maintain the delicate balance between safeguarding your teen's health and allowing the teen the freedom to grow and develop.

EMOTIONAL OBSTACLES
Adolescents who've undergone organ transplants have their own emotional challenges. On top of the usual teenage issues — identity, peer pressure, self-esteem — they may experience fear, anxiety or resentment related to their health, which may impact how they care

for themselves. They may feel like they don't fit in with their peers, which can be both isolating and frustrating.

- **"I hate being different!"** Scars from surgery, the lifelong need for medication and regular checkups, and unwelcome physical changes such as acne or weight gain from antirejection medications can lead to self-consciousness or embarrassment. Adolescence is often a period of heightened awareness of appearances. Feeling "different" can trigger or worsen insecurities.
- **"I'm scared something is going to happen."** The possibility of organ rejection or failure can loom large over an adolescent transplant recipient, creating anxiety or feelings of hopelessness about the future. Your teen may be more likely to have mood swings, avoid conversations about health or even be in denial about health issues.
- **"I don't like being constantly monitored."** Adolescents naturally look for ways to be independent, but a chronic health condition can make them feel like every move and decision they make is being watched. Feeling restricted can lead to resentment toward the situation — and sometimes toward you, the caregiver.

To help your teen navigate the transition toward independence, keep the lines of communication open. Validate feelings by acknowledging fears, frustrations or sadness without dismissing them. Teens aren't always eager to talk to their parents or other caregivers. But knowing that a trusted adult is ready to listen and understand can be incredibly reassuring to them. It's also essential to recognize when teens may need professional counseling, especially if depression, anxiety, or withdrawal become a concern. These mental health issues are common in adolescent transplant recipients, and they can jeopardize transplant care. If you notice this behavior in your teen, contact the transplant team immediately for assistance. The team likely has helped other teens through similar challenges.

BALANCING INDEPENDENCE AND MEDICAL NEEDS
Greater independence is a critical developmental milestone for adolescents. This can sometimes be tricky when they have lifelong medical needs that require at least some oversight.

Taking medicines on time, attending medical appointments and strictly following lifestyle guidelines are musts. But fostering independence is crucial too. And teens may be inclined to exert their autonomy with risky behavior, such as skipping a dose of their medications or not following dietary restrictions. To help avoid such behavior, consider:

- **Teaching the "why" behind the rules.** Teens may resist rules when they don't understand the purpose. Explain how adhering to medication regimens, checkup schedules and healthy lifestyle choices is vital in protecting the transplanted organ. Make it clear that self-care is about empowerment, not just following orders.
- **Involving adolescents in their care.** Encourage your teen to actively participate early on by asking questions during appointments, such as what a particular medicine does and its possible side effects. If an option, let your teen decide when and how to take the medicine. For example, instead of taking medication at 8 a.m. and 8 p.m., shift it to 9 a.m. and 9 p.m. so that your teen can sleep in or take medication with breakfast, making it easier to remember. Several smartphone apps also can help teens track and remember when to take their medications.
- **Turning to peer support.** Some teens may benefit from connecting with other organ transplant recipients who "get it." Support groups for adolescents can provide a sense of belonging and validation, reducing feelings of isolation. Your teen's transplant care team can help connect you with support services.

Involving your teen in healthcare decisions can help develop a sense of ownership over body and well-being. Sometimes, your teen won't do what's asked, and it can feel like you've taken a step backward. But remember, it's all part of the process as your teen tests independence and learns to juggle more responsibility. Remain positive and ready to help get things back on track. Turn occasional stumbles into teachable moments to help build good habits and accountability without adding pressure or guilt.

SOCIAL SITUATIONS

For adolescents, social interactions are essential. Friendships, social activities and extracurricular involvement are critical to their development. However, it's easy for transplant recipients to feel out of place or different, particularly if they tire more quickly than their peers, aren't able to eat certain foods at a party, or can't participate in the same activities others can.

As a parent, you can help your teen navigate social situations in a way that allows the teen to enjoy a fulfilling, connected life while protecting health. The following may help your teen feel more comfortable:

- **Educate peers.** If your teen is comfortable with giving a short explanation about the health situation, decide on a few words to use about the surgery when around peers. "My [organ] wasn't healthy, so it had to be replaced," or something similar. This will usually satisfy curiosity.
- **Lean on a friend.** Your teen may want to consider sharing the transplant story more in-depth with a close friend. This person can help support your teen in social situations and help navigate uncomfortable situations in which saying no is necessary. For example, the friend may decline to participate in a tackle football game or turn down an offer of alcohol.
- **Find activities that focus on strengths.** Encourage your teen to participate in activities that boost self-confidence and make connections with people who share similar interests. Options may be activities such as an art or music class, a noncontact sport, or a drama or engineering club.
- **Aim for comfortable.** For some teens, a small gathering or a get-together at your house is more relaxing and offers more control. Activities such as going to a movie also can be relaxing.

Balance is key. While health is a priority, your teen needs a social life to thrive emotionally. Support friendships, sports and hobbies, even if adjustments are necessary. Help your teen find safe ways to enjoy typical adolescent experiences so that life doesn't feel defined solely by the medical condition.

SCHOOL

Some teens have trouble balancing academic responsibilities with their medical needs. Fatigue and illness, medical appointments, and hospital stays can interfere with their education. A support system can help ease your teen back into the school routine.

- **Work with teachers and school counselors.** They can help create a plan for your teen to handle absences and missed schoolwork. For example, a 504 plan, an individualized education plan (IEP) or an individualized health plan (IHP) addresses necessary accommodations for your teen to thrive, such as extensions on homework and additional time to take tests.
- **Consider limitations.** While it's great to encourage your teen to stay engaged in education and extracurricular activities, some days may be more challenging than others. It's OK to take breaks when needed so that your teen can keep going.

Education is important. However, your teen's physical and emotional well-being should always come first. Remind your teen that it's OK to adjust academic or extracurricular goals to prioritize health.

Handling risky behaviors

Teen parties and social gatherings may involve alcohol, drugs, and smoking or vaping, and your teen will likely face peer pressure to engage in these at some point. Such activities can be dangerous for any adolescent, but for transplant recipients, there are added layers of risk. Therefore, it's important to address these risks early on.

Health consequences

Be upfront with your teen about the possible effects of alcohol, tobacco and drugs. Discuss how they can interfere with the medications your teen takes, increasing the risk of complications or organ rejection.

Also discuss how many drugs have substances added to them, making them even riskier. Injected drugs increase the risk of exposure to many contagious diseases. And if your teen ever needs another transplant, actively using illegal drugs can limit eligibility to receive another organ.

Peer pressure

Equip your teen with strategies for navigating social pressure. This might include talking with your teen ahead of time about polite or humorous ways to refuse drugs or alcohol.

Many teens will still try alcohol and drugs, knowing the risks. Let your teen know that you are always available to talk about any issues in your teen's life, including questions about drinking and tobacco or drug use.

If your teen is having trouble and not adhering to the medication schedule, you'll need to step in. Alert your teen's transplant team, who will likely arrange a visit for your teen to meet with transplant team members. The team also can refer you to a mental health specialist to help you find ways to address the problem.

SEXUAL HEALTH

Sexual health also is an important topic to discuss with any teen. Two concerns stand out:

Sexually transmitted infections

The antirejection medications transplant recipients take make them more vulnerable to infections, including sexually transmitted infections (STIs). STIs include infections such as syphilis, gonorrhea and chlamydia. Discuss with your teen the need to practice safe sex, including condom use, to reduce infection risk.

Birth control

Your teen should discuss the safest form of birth control with a healthcare professional. With some types of birth control, there's an increased risk of blood clots, as well as a reduction in bone density, which is already a potential complication for kidney transplant recipients.

Some antirejection medications can interfere with the effectiveness of birth control pills. Plus, common antirejection medicines such as mycophenolate mofetil (CellCept, Myhibbin) can cause severe birth defects.

Because an unplanned pregnancy can be unsafe to a young transplant recipient and can expose a fetus to potentially harmful medicines, your teen's transplant team may have additional recommendations for birth control and pregnancy prevention.

Don't be surprised if the transplant team wants to speak with your teen separately from you for such discussions. Your teen also may request that you not be in the room. This is typical and gives your teen some privacy to discuss topics that may be embarrassing. It's also a good opportunity for your teen to learn to speak openly with a healthcare professional.

TRANSITIONING TO ADULT CARE

One of the most important responsibilities of parenting an adolescent transplant recipient is preparing the teen for the eventual transition to adult care. Work with your child's transplant team to identify healthcare professionals who have experience with transplant recipients. A smooth handoff from a pediatric team to an adult transplant program is essential for continuity in care.

This transition is a time when older teens will take on even more responsibility for managing their own health. This can be overwhelming for both parents and teens, but it also can be positive and empowering.

- **Start early.** Your child's transplant team can recommend the best time to begin shifting responsibilities from yourself to your child. Every child is different. Some may be ready to take on tasks early, while others may need more time. Discussions about transitioning to adult care may start as early as age 11 or, if your child is older, soon after your child's transplant. Depending on your child's transplant center, the shift to adult care may include a transition clinic or other adolescent services.
- **Add responsibilities.** Once your teen is consistently carrying out a task without needing a reminder, add on another task. In the beginning, you'll probably need to remind your teen to complete the task, such as remembering to take medications without being told. Apps, alarms and pill cases can help with this. You also might have your teen begin scheduling and managing their own appointments.
- **Build practical skills.** Your teen will need to learn and understand how to navigate adult healthcare successfully. Older teens might

be shown how to budget for medicine and deductibles, get tips on organizing health records, and learn how health insurance works.

- **Prepare for college life.** Teens going away to college should reach out to the transplant team for suggestions on transplant resources close to their schools. Your teen can set up a meeting with a nearby transplant center before starting college. It's also a good idea to find a pharmacy near the college to handle all prescriptions. Also touch base with the college to ensure your teen receives any necessary accommodations.

Like all humans, your teen is likely to make mistakes. That's typical. Most young transplant recipients won't completely master self-management till they're in their 20s. Even as they approach young adulthood, they may need you to serve as a backup and continue offering reminders as needed.

Though it can be tempting to intervene more frequently, this is a necessary step toward independence. The transition period is a unique time when your teen gets ample support from you and the pediatric care team while learning and gaining the confidence and skills typically needed to manage care in the near future.

Offer support but let your teen take the lead when it comes to communicating with healthcare professionals and managing health. When transplant recipients turn 18, they're legally considered adults, so the transplant care team will need permission from your teen to talk about health matters with you.

Your next chapter

Recovering from transplant surgery can stir up a mix of emotions — excitement, relief and sometimes anxiety. As you begin this new chapter in your life, it's natural to feel uncertain about what lies ahead. These emotions are common and completely valid. At the same time, you also may find that life is more at ease without your previous stresses. You no longer have to wait for the transplant call.

With a healthy, functioning organ, you'll likely experience more energy and freedom and the ability to do things that were once difficult or out of reach. In time — and with the approval of your transplant team — you may find yourself enjoying long walks, cooking meals, returning to school or work, driving again, and reconnecting with favorite activities. You'll gradually build more independence and settle into a routine that fits your new normal, all while exercising caution and remaining vigilant.

The first few months can be demanding, both physically and emotionally. But over time, your strength, mood and overall well-being are expected to improve. Staying positive, flexible and proactive — especially by having a plan for managing challenges — can make a big difference in your recovery. Active coping is linked to better quality of life in transplant patients.

Organ transplantation is one of the greatest achievements of modern medicine. It's a life-changing gift that reflects the power of science, the generosity of others, and the resilience of the human body and spirit. It's a second chance at life — not just to survive but to truly live.

Additional resources

Air Care Alliance
www.aircarealliance.org
Maintains a list of known agencies that provide free air service for patient transport.

Air Charity Network
https://aircharitynetwork.org
877-621-7177
Provides free transport services for patients with documented medical and financial needs using private pilots and their aircraft.

American Kidney Fund
www.kidneyfund.org/kidney-donation-and-transplant/transplant
-waiting-list
Maintains a list of people in the United States who need a kidney transplant and want to be matched with an organ from a deceased donor. The list is managed by UNOS.

American Liver Foundation
www.liverfoundation.org
info@liverfoundation.org
800-465-4837
Provides current news and information on liver-related topics, helping patients, friends and families affected by liver disease.

American Society of Transplantation

www.myast.org

856-439-9986

Dedicated to advancing the field of transplantation and improving care by promoting research, education, advocacy and organ donation.

- Living kidney donor toolkit: www.livingdonortoolkit.com/medical -toolkit
- Living liver donor toolkit: www.livingdonortoolkit.com/living-liver -medical-toolkit

Angel Flight

www.angelflight.com

918-749-8992

Provides free air transportation on private aircraft for people not able to afford the service on their own.

Association of Organ Procurement Organizations

www.aopo.org

703-556-4242

Leader in organ donation and transplantation through continual improvement of the donation process, collaboration with stakeholders and sharing of best practices.

Children's Health Insurance Program (CHIP)

www.healthcare.gov/medicaid-chip/childrens-health-insurance-program/

800-318-2596

Provides low-cost health coverage to children in families that earn too much money to qualify for Medicaid.

Children's Organ Transplant Association (COTA)

https://cota.org

800-366-2682

Helps overcome financial barriers to a lifesaving transplant by providing fundraising assistance and family support.

Donate Life America
https://donatelife.net
Nonprofit organization working to increase the number of donated organs, eyes and tissues available to save and heal lives.

Donor Network of Arizona
www.dnaz.org
Nonprofit organ procurement organization in Arizona that saves lives through organ, eye and tissue donation.

Enduring Hearts
www.enduringhearts.org
Supports research to increase longevity and improve quality of life for children with transplanted hearts.

Gift of Life Transplant House
https://gift-of-life.org
office@gift-of-life.org
507-288-7470
Home away from home in Rochester, Minnesota, to serve transplant patients and their families, benefiting the health and well-being of all.

GiveForward
www.giveforward.com
Information for families on how to create individual fundraising pages for loved ones facing a medical crisis.

Health Insurance Marketplace
www.healthcare.gov
800-318-2596
Provides information on existing regulations and policies and health insurance options under the Affordable Care Act.

Help Hope Live
www.helphopelive.org
support@helphopelive.org
800-642-8399

Supports community-based fundraising for people with unmet medical expenses and related costs due to cell and organ transplants or catastrophic injuries and illnesses.

Health Resources & Services Administration
www.organdonor.gov
Provides outreach to educate the public and encourage more people to register as organ, eye and tissue donors.

Kidney Paired Donation
https://unos.org/transplant/kidney-paired-donation/
A pilot project of OPTN that provides kidney transplant candidates another option to receive an organ. Living-donor kidneys are swapped so each recipient receives a compatible match.

LifeSource
www.life-source.org
First responders who specialize in the process of organ donation, see that transplants reach waiting recipients, support donor families and inspire people to register as donors.

LifeQuest Organ Recovery Services
https://lifequestfla.org
Nonprofit organ procurement organization in Florida that saves lives through organ, eye and tissue donation.

Lung Transplant Foundation
https://lungtransplantfoundation.org
Information and resources to improve the lives of lung transplant recipients and their families.

Mayo Clinic
www.MayoClinic.org
Mayo Clinic's online health information portal.

Mayo Clinic Connect
https://connect.mayoclinic.org
An online community moderated by Mayo Clinic where patients and caregivers can share experiences, find support, and connect with others facing similar health challenges.

Mayo Clinic Transplant on Facebook
www.facebook.com/MayoClinicTransplant
Community of transplant recipients and educators who share information on transplantation at Mayo Clinic.

Medicare
www.medicare.gov/coverage/organ-transplants#
The U.S. government's health insurance program for people age 65 and older and younger people with disabilities.

National Alliance for Caregiving
www.caregiving.org
Dedicated to research, advocacy and innovation to make life better for family caregivers.

National Kidney Foundation
www.kidney.org
Resource for information about kidney transplantation.

National Kidney Registry
www.kidneyregistry.com
Dedicated to increasing living kidney donation, ensuring better donor-recipient matches, and providing comprehensive support and protections for living donors.

National Living Donor Assistance Center
www.livingdonorassistance.org
A nationwide system that provides reimbursement of travel and subsistence expenses, lost wages, and dependent care expenses to people being evaluated for or undergoing living organ donation.

National Minority Organ Tissue Transplant Education Program (MOTTEP)

www.natlmottep.org

202-865-4888

Information on organ tissue transplants for Black Americans.

Organ Procurement and Transplant Network (OPTN)

https://optn.transplant.hrsa.gov

A unique public-private partnership that links all professionals involved in the U.S. organ donation and transplantation system.

Organ Transplant Support

www.organtransplantsupport.org

Provides education, support and resources for transplant families and promotes organ and tissue donor awareness.

OurLegacy

https://www.ourlegacyfl.org

Nonprofit organ procurement organization in Florida that saves lives through organ, eye and tissue donation.

Patient Advocate Foundation

www.patientadvocate.org

A nonprofit organization that provides case management services and financial aid to people with chronic, life-threatening and debilitating illnesses.

Scientific Registry of Transplant Recipients

www.srtr.org

Supports the transplant community with analyses in an effort to achieve better results and experiences.

Today's Caregiver

https://caregiver.com

Leading provider of information, support and guidance for family and professional caregivers.

Trio
www.trioweb.org
An independent not-for-profit international organization committed to improving the quality of life for transplant candidates, transplant recipients and involved families.

United Network for Organ Sharing (UNOS)
https://unos.org
Manages the waiting list for a transplant in the U.S. and matches donors to recipients.

Index

antirejection medications (*continued*)

modified cyclosporine (Neoral, Gengraf), 184, 195

mycophenolate mofetil (Cell-Cept, Myhibbin), 164, 184, 193, 232, 256

mycophenolic sodium (Myfortic), 184, 193, 232

prednisone, 164, 184, 185, 187, 192, 219, 220, 239

pregnancy and, 232–233

purpose of, 166, 183

sirolimus (Rapamune), 164, 184, 186, 194–195, 219

skin care and, 219, 220–221

sun care and, 226–227

tacrolimus (Prograf, Astagraf XL, Envarsus XR), 164, 184, 186, 193–194, 222

types of, 164, 184

vaccinations and, 240

antirejection medications, side effects of, 32, 164–165, 183, 184, 187

of azathioprine, 195

in children, 244–245

of cyclosporine and modified cyclosporine, 195

medications to treat, 187–189

of mycophenolate mofetil and mycophenolic sodium, 193

of prednisone and methylpred-nisolone, 192

of sirolimus, 194–195

of tacrolimus, 193–194

Association of Organ Procurement Organizations, 261

Astagraf XL (tacrolimus), 164, 184, 186, 193–194, 222

autoimmune conditions, 14, 15, 68, 74, 156

Azasan (azathioprine), 184, 195

azathioprine (Imuran, Azasan), 184, 195

B

bags, packing

caregiver bags, 143

recipient's extended-stay bag, 142

recipient's hospital bag, 141–142

biliary atresia, 20, 73, 172

bioartificial livers, 84–85

bioengineering, 84–85, 87

blood pressure. *See also* high blood pressure; low blood pressure

changes in, 193, 210

home monitoring of, 139, 211

ideal readings, 211

medications to control, 182, 184, 186, 187, 244

organ rejection and, 198

when to call your care team, 210

bone marrow transplant, 26, 91

bowel transplant. *See* small intestine transplant

bronchiolitis obliterans, 73

C

call, getting the. *See* transplant call

candidate evaluation. *See* transplant candidate evaluation

cannabis, 229

cardiomyopathy, 17, 70, 216

cardiopulmonary stress test, 41

donor advocates, 91, 98
donor family, contacting, 230–231
Donor Network of Arizona, 262
donors, types of, 78–79. See also
living-donor transplants
dry runs, 131, 138–140

E

eating out after surgery, 225, 226
Ebers Papyrus, 10
emphysema, 21
Enduring Hearts, 262
Envarsus XR (tacrolimus), 164, 184,
186, 193–194, 222
estimated glomerular filtration rate
(eGFR), 38–39
estimated post-transplant survival
(EPTS) score, 39–40, 83
everolimus (Afinitor, Zortress), 164,
184
extracorporeal membrane oxygenation (ECMO), 71, 152
ex vivo lung perfusion (EVLP), 80–81

F

face transplant, 24–25
Family and Medical Leave Act
(FMLA), 97, 130
finances. See costs and finances
focal glomerulosclerosis, 68
food safety, 201–205, 225, 226
fungal infections, 183, 189, 222,
223, 229, 244

G

genetic conditions, 20, 21, 68, 74, 76
genetic engineering, 87

Gengraf (modified cyclosporine),
184, 195
Gift of Life Transplant House, 262
GiveForward, 262
glomerular filtration rate (GFR),
38–39

H

hair care after surgery, 222–223
hand transplant, 24–25
health inequities, 38–39, 86
health insurance, 51–53
Children's Health Insurance
Program (CHIP), 129, 261
Medicaid, 129, 261
Medicare, 51–52, 54, 56, 264
Medigap policy, 51–52
patient advocates and, 53
private insurance, 51
Health Insurance Marketplace,
262
Health Resources & Services
Administration, 263
heart arrhythmias, 71
heart catheterization, 41
heart defects, 17, 28
heart failure, 17–18, 28–29, 40, 44,
70
heart-kidney transplant, 47
heart-liver transplant, 47
heart-lung machine, 151, 152, 174,
176
heart-lung transplant, 22, 47
heart transplant, 10, 17–18, 28–29
in children, 70–71, 175
evaluation and testing for,
40–41
surgery, 150–152
Heimbach, Julie K., 44–45

liver disease and liver failure, 19
  alcohol-associated liver disease,
    20, 43
  awareness campaigns, 172
  bioartificial livers and, 84–85
  in children, 72, 73, 74
  cirrhosis (chronic liver disease),
    20, 42–43, 74, 139, 156
  as complication of intestinal
    transplant, 73
  liver transplants and, 72
  metabolic liver diseases, 73
  Model for End-Stage Liver
    Disease (MELD) score,
    44–46, 74, 75, 83
  Pediatric End-Stage Liver
    Disease (PELD) score, 74, 75
  primary biliary cirrhosis, 156
  resources, 260
  steatotic liver disease (formerly
    fatty liver disease), 19, 20, 43,
    44
liver-kidney transplant, 47
liver transplant, 10, 19–20
  in children, 72–75, 172–173,
    175–177
  evaluation and testing for, 42–46
  living-donor considerations and
    requirements, 92–93
  living-donor transplants, 13, 74–75,
    79, 105, 146, 148, 150, 175
  obesity and, 44–45
  sleeve gastrectomy combined
    with, 44–45
  surgery, 148–150, 152–153,
    156–158
  wait times for livers, 109
living-donor transplants, 88–90
  benefits to recipients, 40, 61, 75,
    83, 90

  for children, 69, 72, 74–75
  directed donation, 90
  donation chains, 95, 96
  donor advocates for, 98
  donor and recipient costs, 94–97
  donor considerations, 97
  donor evaluation process, 98–100
  donor requirements, 90–95
  insurance coverage for, 52
  intestinal transplants, 72, 73
  kidney donation surgery, 101–103
  kidney donor considerations and
    requirements, 93–94
  kidney transplants, 34, 52, 69,
    77, 79, 88–90, 91, 93–97
  liver donation surgery and
    recovery, 101, 104, 105
  liver donor considerations and
    requirements, 92–93
  liver transplants, 13, 74–75, 79,
    105, 146, 148, 150, 175
  nondirected donation, 88–90
  organs suitable for, 66
  paired donations, 69, 77, 84–85,
    92, 94, 95, 263
  preemptive kidney transplants, 69
  recovery from and life after
    donation surgery, 103–107
  resources, 261, 263, 264
  statistics, 79
  talking to friends and family
    about, 118–119
low blood pressure, 42, 68, 198
**lung Composite Allocation Score
  (CAS),** 41
lung disease, 21, 73, 92, 94
lung transplant, 10, 20–22
  in children, 73, 176
  double-lung transplants, 22, 152,
    153, 155

evaluation and testing for, 41–42
single-lung transplants, 22, 152, 153

Lung Transplant Foundation, 263

M

marijuana, 229
Mayo Clinic, 263
Mayo Clinic Connect, 264
Mayo Clinic Transplant on Face-book, 264
Medicaid, 129, 261
Medicare, 51–52, 54, 56, 264
medication. *See also* antirejection medications
    after surgery, 162–165
    antifungal medicines, 182, 183, 189, 222, 224
    caregiver tips for managing, 196
    costs of, 53–54, 57
    managing regimens, 189–192
Medigap policies, 51–52
Medrol (methylprednisolone), 184, 192
methylprednisolone (Medrol, Solu-Medrol), 184, 192
Model for End-Stage Liver Disease (MELD) score, 44–46, 74, 75, 83
modified cyclosporine (Neoral, Gengraf), 184, 195
multiorgan transplants, 22, 47
mycophenolate mofetil (CellCept, Myhibbin), 164, 184, 193, 232, 256
mycophenolic sodium (Myfortic), 184, 193, 232
Myfortic (mycophenolic sodium), 184, 193, 232

Myhibbin (mycophenolate mofetil), 164, 184, 193, 232, 256

N

nail care after surgery, 223, 224
National Alliance for Caregiving, 264
National Kidney Foundation, 264
National Kidney Registry, 264
National Living Donor Assistance Center, 264
National Minority Organ Tissue Transplant Education Program (MOTTEP), 265
Neoral (modified cyclosporine), 184, 195
nephrotic syndrome, 68
nondirected donation, 88–90

O

obesity, 44–45
oligomeganephronia, 60
operating room. *See* surgery
organizations. *See* transplant organizations
organ procurement, 136–137
Organ Procurement and Transplant Network (OPTN), 9–10, 36, 79, 265
    kidney transplant allocation scoring process, 40
    multiple hospital listings, 84
    transplant waitlist, 130
    United Network for Organ Sharing and, 82
organ procurement organizations (OPOs), 37, 82, 109, 131, 230–231

V

ventricular assist device (VAD), 71
vesicoureteral reflux, 17

W

waitlists, 108–110
    caregiver roles while on,
        121–123
    children on, 125
    choosing support groups while
        on, 116
    getting listed, 82–83
    listing at multiple hospitals, 84
    parental roles while children are
        on, 124–132

staying organized while on, 117,
    120–121
talking to friends and family
    while on, 118–119
your mental well-being while on,
    112–117
your physical health while on,
    110–112
Wilson's disease, 20, 73

X

xenotransplantation, 87

Z

Zortress (everolimus), 164, 184

Scan to learn more about
Mayo Clinic's transplant programs

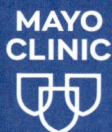

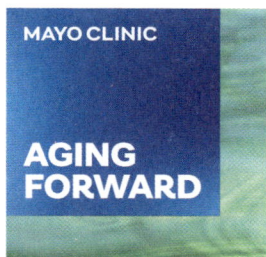

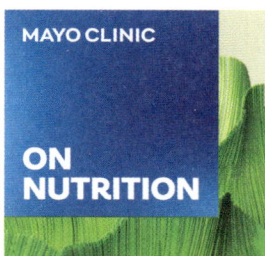

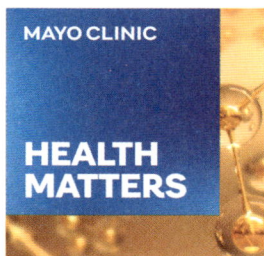

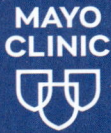

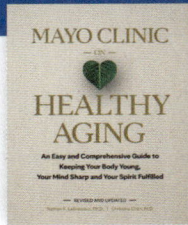

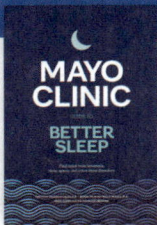

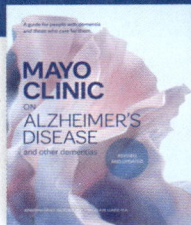

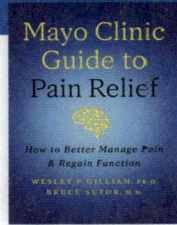